YET
WILL
I
PRAISE
HIM

"In her book, *Yet Will I Praise Him: Living and Parenting with a Chronic Illness,* Hannah Wingert articulates the struggles and emotions plagued by chronic illness warriors; words often difficult to express. Her words ring true. Readers will exclaim, "She gets me!"

Hannah Wingert is a superhero of faith with chronic illness. She possesses the unique faith filled perspective of parenting children with chronic illnesses while battling an illness herself. Give this woman a cape!"

—April Dawn White,
co-author of *Destination Hope* (releasing spring 2021)

"Hannah gives a realistic look at what it is like being a chronically ill mom and what being a parent of chronically ill children entails. *Yet Will I Praise Him* is an inspirational book for those in similar walks of life and an informative book for those who yearn to understand more about what it takes to live with a chronic illness."

—Daphne Self,
author of *Journey On: Through This Shadowed Valley*

YET WILL I PRAISE HIM

LIVING AND PARENTING WITH A CHRONIC ILLNESS

Hannah Wingert

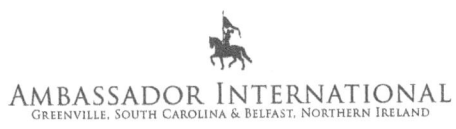

AMBASSADOR INTERNATIONAL
GREENVILLE, SOUTH CAROLINA & BELFAST, NORTHERN IRELAND
www.ambassador-international.com

Yet Will I Praise Him
Living and Parenting With A Chronic Illness
©2020 by Hannah Wingert

All rights reserved

ISBN: 978-1-64960-011-0
eISBN: 978-1-64960-012-7
Library of Congress Control Number: 2020949345

Cover Design by Kim Bolton
Interior Typesetting by Hannah Nichols
Digital edition by Anna Riebe Raats

Unless otherwise marked, Scripture quotations are from The ESV® Bible (The Holy Bible, English Standard Version®), copyright © 2001 by Crossway, a publishing ministry of Good News Publishers. Used by permission. All rights reserved.

Scripture marked NKJV taken from the New King James Version®. Copyright © 1982 by Thomas Nelson. Used by permission. All rights reserved.

Scripture marked KJV taken from the King James Version. Public Domain.

AMBASSADOR INTERNATIONAL
Emerald House
411 University Ridge, Suite B14
Greenville, SC 29601, USA
www.ambassador-international.com

AMBASSADOR BOOKS
The Mount
2 Woodstock Link
Belfast, BT6 8DD, Northern Ireland, UK
www.ambassadormedia.co.uk

The colophon is a trademark of Ambassador, a Christian publishing company.

Dedicated to my children, Katie, Nate, Anna, and Davy. Thank you for teaching me how to find the joy in life no matter what it throws at me.

CONTENTS

ABOUT THIS BOOK   11

PREFACE   13

INTRODUCTION
WHAT IS A SPOONIE?   17

PART ONE
LIVING AS A SPOONIE   21

CHAPTER ONE
IF GOD IS GOOD, WHY DOESN'T HE HEAL ME?   23

CHAPTER TWO
WHAT YOU CAN LEARN FROM YOUR CHRONIC ILLNESS   33

CHAPTER THREE
DOES GOD GIVE YOU MORE THAN YOU CAN HANDLE?   43

CHAPTER FOUR
COPING AS A SPOONIE   49

CHAPTER FIVE
THE FIVE STAGES OF GRIEF FOR SPOONIES   55

CHAPTER SIX
WHAT TO DO WHEN THE GUILT HITS   67

CHAPTER SEVEN
HOW A CHRONIC ILLNESS AFFECTS YOUR SPOUSE   71

CHAPTER EIGHT
LIFE AS A SPOONIE DAD   85

PART TWO
PARENTING AS A SPOONIE   99

CHAPTER NINE
WHAT YOUR KIDS CAN LEARN FROM YOUR CHRONIC ILLNESS   101

CHAPTER TEN
WHEN YOU AND YOUR CHILD(REN) ARE SPOONIES   111

CHAPTER ELEVEN
PREPPING FOR MEDICAL APPOINTMENTS   129

CHAPTER TWELVE
PARENTING FROM THE COUCH   137

CHAPTER THIRTEEN
HOUSEKEEPING HACKS   147

CHAPTER FOURTEEN
LIFE HACKS   161

PART THREE
LOVING A SPOONIE   169

CHAPTER FIFTEEN
TO THE SPOUSE OF A SPOONIE   171

CHAPTER SIXTEEN
WHAT NOT TO SAY TO A SPOONIE PARENT (AND WHAT TO SAY INSTEAD)   183

CONCLUSION   195

RESOURCES   197

ABOUT THE AUTHOR   199

Why art thou cast down, O my soul? and why art thou disquieted within me? hope in God: for I shall yet praise him, who is the health of my countenance, and my God.

Psalm 43:5 KJV

ABOUT THIS BOOK

THIS BOOK DOES NOT HAVE to be read cover to cover. Pick a chapter that covers something you're dealing with right now, or just read a section from that chapter. You can read the chapters out of order, and there is also a chapter wrap-up at the end of each one that you can skim through when you're running short on time or spoons. Enjoy!

PREFACE

I'VE ALWAYS KNOWN THERE WAS something different about me. Growing up, I had weird aches and pains that didn't make much sense. I got tired easily, frequently had stomach issues, and hated being in the sun because it made me feel sick and gave me headaches. In contrast, my four siblings had seemingly endless energy and never complained of pain. By the time I was a teenager, I often requested to push the shopping cart while I was out with my family because, after just a short time of walking, my legs would feel like jelly and give out with no warning. Doctor after doctor dismissed my complaints, and I convinced myself that I was just being a wimp.

When I started having kids, my health began to go downhill fast. The first pregnancy wasn't too bad, but I never really recovered from the second one. And then I had two more, back to back, with only seven months in between them, and my body *really* started to fall apart. By the end of each one of those last two pregnancies, I was in incredible pain, had no energy, and could barely walk. I was so miserable at the end of the pregnancy with my last baby that I begged my doctor to induce me before my due date. He refused, but thankfully, my little Davy must have realized that Mama just couldn't do it anymore and decided to make his debut two days after my due date, a far cry from his three older siblings who were one to two weeks late.

I'm not sure if it was because the last two pregnancies were so close together or because Davy's infancy was so stressful for me due to his medical complexity, but after he was born, my health began to decline rapidly. I had problems with my legs buckling, was in constant pain, and had fatigue so severe that I could barely talk sometimes, but I chalked it up to the stress of having a baby with special needs.

Sweet little Davy's first year was intensely hard for him and our whole family. He screamed like he was in horrible pain whenever I tried to feed him and, by the time he was two months old, we were signing consent forms to have a feeding tube surgically placed in his precious little tummy so he could get the nutrition he needed to grow. Davy was diagnosed with hypotonia, reflux, chronic lung infections, tracheomalacia, developmental delays, and more, and he was absolutely miserable most of the time. I spent his first year of life in the hospital and at doctors' appointments with him, often holding him down for medical tests that would inevitably come back normal again, leaving us with no answers. Davy screamed almost constantly and was so sensitive to stimulation that he couldn't even handle having his older siblings near him at times. I had perpetual bruises on both of my forearms from trying to hold him while he arched his back and screamed in my arms, but if I put him down, he screamed even harder and turned blue.

As he grew, Davy slowly but surely started doing better, and our lives got easier and less stressful. When he was around a year old, we switched to a new health system with all new doctors for his care, and at one of the first appointments with his new geneticist, she diagnosed him with an unspecified connective tissue disorder, giving us the start of answers to the questions that plagued us. He had his G-Tube removed at the age of eighteen months because he was eating one hundred percent of his food by mouth.

Now that things had settled down a little with Davy, I decided that it was time to figure out what was going on with me now. The experience I'd gained on how to research and present information to Davy's doctors during my search to figure out what was wrong with my baby could now be used for questions about my own health. For years, I'd asked doctors about just one or two of my weird symptoms at a time, but now I knew that I had to take a different approach. I flipped to the back of the worn college-ruled notebook I'd used to document and chart Davy's life so far and started writing down all my symptoms and random issues. Two pages later, I was done and ready for battle. At my appointment later that month, I handed the list to my primary care doctor, and her jaw dropped. She wasn't sure where to start so she referred me to a neurologist who ran some tests that all came back normal. The next step was to see a rheumatologist, so I booked the next available appointment and waited. During the four-month wait to see rheumatology, I posted a picture of Davy's hypermobile ankle on Instagram, and someone asked if he had Ehlers Danlos Syndrome. I knew that it was a connective tissue disorder, which we were aware Davy had some type of, so I decided to look into it.

The more research on Ehlers Danlos Syndrome, or EDS, that I did, the more things made sense, not only for Davy but for me as well. It also seemed to fit Davy's older siblings as well although they weren't as severely affected as him.

At Davy's next appointment with his geneticist, I mentioned EDS, and it was like a light went on in the room. When I left her office an hour later, we had both been informally diagnosed with EDS and had appointments scheduled later that summer to formally test and diagnose me along with my three older children. I cried in the elevator down to the parking garage because all of a sudden, my whole life made sense. That day was completely life-changing.

Since then, all four of my kids—Katie, Nate, Anna, Davy—and I have been diagnosed with the hypermobile type of Ehlers Danlos Syndrome or hEDS. Katie, Nate, and Davy also have asthma, eczema, and allergies along with a variety of other diagnoses. I have asthma, eczema, Postural Orthostatic Tachycardia Syndrome or POTS, Eosinophilic Esophagitis or EoE, Mast Cell Activation Disorder or MCAD, and more. Thankfully, Anna doesn't seem to be very affected by her EDS right now although I know that can quickly change without much warning.

Being diagnosed didn't stop me from getting worse, though. I struggle to get through each day, and I know that it's not going to get better. I've had to learn to give myself grace for the bad days and to not push myself too much on the good days. I've had to learn to let go of some things completely and ask for help for others. I've had to grieve the loss of the life that I thought I was going to have.

I hope that this book helps you in your journey as a parent with a chronic illness. While I've written it to moms, I have also included a chapter for chronically ill dads since they're facing a lot of the same challenges.

Hannah

INTRODUCTION
WHAT IS A SPOONIE?

I'M A SPOONIE. AND, IF you're reading this book, you're probably a spoonie, too. Some of you may be doing a fist pump right now (gently, of course! We don't want any injuries), and yelling, "Spoonies, unite!" And some of you may be sitting there scratching your head and thinking, "Wait, is this a cookbook?"

Nope. It's not. You won't find one single recipe in this book. However, I will refer to spoons throughout the chapters so it might be helpful to make sure we're all on the same page as to what that means.

To put it simply, a spoonie is anyone who has a chronic illness or disorder such as Lupus, Fibromyalgia, Ehlers Danlos Syndrome (which is what I have), Multiple Sclerosis, Myalgic Encephalomyelitis, Chronic Fatigue Syndrome, etc.

The term "spoonie" came from The Spoon Theory which was written by lupus sufferer Christine Miserandino from butyoudontlooksick.com. She explained how she was eating out with a friend and was trying to answer her friend's questions about what it's like to have a chronic illness when she was inspired to grab a bunch of spoons from her table and the empty surrounding tables as an illustration.

She handed her friend the handful of spoons and explained that each one represented a unit of energy for the day. Most people have an unlimited supply of spoons each day, but many of those who fight chronic illness must ration theirs. As her friend reviewed her usual daily activities such as getting ready for work, running errands, etc, Christine took away a spoon or two for each one. By dinnertime of her theoretical day, her friend had only one spoon left in her hand, and Christine explained that she now needed to decide if she would use that spoon to cook herself dinner, clean up her house a little, or do something fun because she didn't have enough spoons to do it all. Her friend was stunned at the realization of what it was like to have a chronic illness and was able to understand Christine's life better.

Since Christine first came up with the Spoon Theory, it has taken off in popularity. Some people hate it, but many love how it explains living with a chronic illness in concrete terms. Granted, it doesn't cover all the ins-and-outs of having a chronic illness and everyone's symptoms are different, but it gives healthy people a way to visualize what we go through every day. Using the Spoon Theory, someone in the chronic illness community at some point dubbed us all "spoonies" and the name stuck.

Like most spoonies, I never know how many spoons I'm going to get each day. Some days, I have a whole handful and other days, I just get a few and must plan my day very carefully. Even on the days when I start out with a lot, I have to be aware that they can easily disappear like some kind of bad magic show leaving me with none left to finish the day. Overdoing it often means borrowing spoons from the next few days which can leave me lying on the couch in pain, so fatigued that breathing feels like too much work.

If you're not a fan of the Spoon Theory, another way to explain chronic illness to someone who doesn't have one is by using your phone battery as an example. While most people have a battery that easily lasts them all day, someone with a chronic illness has a battery that runs out quickly and is prone to "energy hogs," i.e. things that sucks the energy out of your battery such as being in an area with poor signal or playing a game that uses lots of data. Resting and taking care of ourselves is how we recharge our batteries, but just to make things even more interesting, our chargers are pretty pathetic, taking over twice as long to recharge the battery than a normal charger would.

Being a spoonie is hard, but you can learn to embrace your spoons and get the most out of them that you can. Acknowledging your limitations and being purposeful with pacing yourself is very important to your well-being, but it won't happen overnight. It's an ongoing process that you'll have to re-learn and go through over and over again. Knowing that can help you deal with it.

INTRODUCTION WRAP-UP

- The Spoon Theory is a good way to explain your chronic illness to others in a way they can understand.
- Using your phone battery as an example also works well.
- How to trust God in the hard times

PART ONE

LIVING AS A SPOONIE

CHAPTER ONE

IF GOD IS GOOD, WHY DOESN'T HE HEAL ME?

THIS IS A QUESTION I'VE struggled with over and over. If God is good, why is there suffering in the world? Why do I have this painful condition and why, why, why do my children have to suffer with it, too? When Davy was struggling so much during his first year of life, I was bitterly angry with God. Why would a good God allow an innocent baby to suffer like that? It wasn't fair.

It took me several years of alternating between being angry at God and begging Him to help before I was finally able to be at peace with the suffering that my kids and I are going through and will continue to experience throughout our whole lives.

It wasn't an easy road, though. It was filled with twists and turns, potholes and wash-outs. I still struggle with those same thoughts sometimes, but I've learned how to handle them better by reminding myself of the truth in God's Word. I want to go over those truths with you in this chapter.

IT ISN'T FAIR

Let's start with one of the most common thoughts . . . it isn't fair. You're right. It isn't fair. You didn't do anything to deserve your chronic illness. It's not fair that you have to push through pain just to make it through a day. It's not fair that your kids have to miss out on activities because you're not well enough to take them. It's not fair that you had to quit the job you love just because your dysfunctional body won't let you do it anymore. But did Jesus deserve to die one of the most torturous deaths known to man? Nope. That wasn't fair either.

The world likes to tell us that we deserve fairness but believing that can lead to a loss of faith because things happen to us that aren't fair. Life isn't fair, and neither is God. If God were fair, He wouldn't allow us to go on living our lives in direct disobedience to Him, and He wouldn't show us the grace that saves us. The book of Matthew reminds us that God does not deal with us according to our sin.

> For He makes His sun rise on the evil and on the good, and sends rain on the just and on the unjust. Matthew 5:45b

IS IT OKAY TO BE ANGRY WITH GOD?

I used to believe it was okay to be angry with God for not healing me or my children. After all, Ephesians 4:26b says, "Be angry and sin not." So, is God telling us that it is okay to be angry? Sure, if it's a righteous anger and not a sinful one. But what's the difference between those two types of anger?

A righteous anger is one that is directed at sin and the twisting of God's Word. It is anger at the injustice of the world and how the innocent suffer because of the sins of others. The goal of righteous anger is a desire to change the situation and help others.

A sinful anger is one that comes from my sin nature. It is demonstrated in rebellion, bitterness, rage, and a lack of self-control. The focus of sinful anger is me and what I want. It's rooted in selfishness and pride and does not care about others.

When I'm angry at God for my chronic illness, it's not a righteous anger. It's not focused on sin in the world, it's focused on what I think is fair for me. Being angry with God is a sin, pure and simple. I'm not saying I don't still feel that way sometimes, but I've learned to recognize it for what it is, and, like any other sin, it must be confessed, and a change made in my behavior.

IS GOD PUNISHING ME FOR SOMETHING?

I don't believe that God necessarily gives us trials, but I do believe that He allows us to go through them for our benefit and growth. Our pain and struggles are a direct result of living in a broken, sinful world. Now, that doesn't mean that your chronic illness was caused by you sinning at some point and it doesn't mean that it was caused by someone else's sin either. This world is imperfect, and our bodies are imperfect. Between sin in the world and imperfections, we will have struggles. Period. Everyone does at some point in their life and in different ways.

On a more scientific level, think about Adam and Eve. God created them with perfect DNA and perfect bodies. Let us say you paint a beautiful picture that's completely perfect. Someone takes that picture and copies it on a copy machine, and then someone else makes a copy of the copy and someone else makes a copy of the copy and so on. Each time a copy is made from the previous one, the picture will develop more and more tiny, microscopic imperfections until eventually, it's blurry and barely resembles the original. Our DNA and bodies are the same way. With continued copying onto the next generation, they break down and change from what they originally were. That is why Adam and Eve's children could marry their siblings. Their DNA was still perfect, but over time, genetic variations have made it so that marrying a relative now can have adverse effects on the children of that union. The increased number of genetic syndromes and health problems, as well as the higher numbers of people affected, are a result of the brokenness and imperfection of the world we live in.

WHAT IS THE PURPOSE OF MY CHRONIC ILLNESS?

You may not be able to see the purpose behind your chronic illness right now. In fact, you may never see it in your lifetime, but rest assured that God has a purpose for it and for you. In 2 Corinthians, Paul says, "Three times I pleaded with the Lord about this, that it should leave me. But He said to me,

My grace is sufficient for you, for My power is made perfect in weakness. Therefore I will boast all the more gladly of my weaknesses, so that the power of Christ may rest upon me."

We don't know what Paul suffered from, but he alluded to it several times in his writings. Whatever it was, he begged God to take it from him just as you have probably done with your chronic illness. But God chose not to heal him, and we can see why now. Paul's suffering has encouraged countless believers who are going through their own trials. It demonstrates that God can use your weakness as a strength, and it shows us how to rely more fully on God's power instead of our own. Paul may never have known exactly how his health problem would work in the lives of others, but God knew. God sees the whole timeline from the beginning to the end. We see only a small portion of it which means that we may never know the purpose behind our pain, but we can rest assured that He has one.

If you let it, your chronic illness can help you rely more on God each day. It can help you turn your eyes heavenward instead of focusing on the things of this world. It can remind you of how Jesus suffered for your sins so that you could be saved. That thought right there blows me away . . . Jesus can relate to my pain because He suffered, too.

Your chronic illness can also touch other people's lives. It can help you relate to others so that you can encourage them and give them the opportunity to be a blessing to you, which in return, blesses them. Keeping your eyes on Jesus and letting Him shine through you even when you're in constant pain can speak louder to others than any sermon could.

I know a sweet lady who spent years bent over in a wheelchair unable to straighten her body and in such excruciating pain that not even the strongest pain medication could touch it. Ema McKinley's family attended my church and so I grew up hearing about her accident at work that left her with severe Complex Regional Pain Syndrome or CRPS as a result. On Christmas Eve night, over eighteen years after her accident, she experienced an amazing miracle where she literally felt Jesus pick her up off the floor where she had fallen and heal her body. The next morning, her sons arrived at her house to celebrate Christmas with her and were completely blown away to see their mother standing straight and walking—things she hadn't been able to do in years. Why am I telling you about this? Because the beauty and miracle in her story (which you can read in her book, *Rush of Heaven*) is not in her healing. It's in the years before her healing when she was unable to care for herself, sit up straight, or relieve her pain at all no matter what was prescribed to her. During that time, she never lost her faith in God. She trusted Him no matter what, even though she knew she would probably spend the rest of her life like that. She used that time and her condition to encourage and point others to Christ. She continued to believe in God's goodness and His mercy.

HOW CAN I FIND COMFORT FOR MY CHRONIC ILLNESS?

I've begged God to heal me from my EDS and all of the other conditions that go along with it, but He has not chosen to do so. Instead of healing, He offers me comfort and I can choose to accept or reject it. God's comfort comes from the Bible, and it can come from others as well.

I can find comfort in the knowledge that someday, I will be with Christ and will not be in pain anymore.

> He will wipe away every tear from their eyes, and death shall be no more, neither shall there be mourning, nor crying, nor pain anymore, for the former things have passed away. Revelation 21:4

But for now, I'm here on earth with my earthly body and all of its imperfections and disabilities. So, while that verse gives me comfort for the future, it doesn't necessarily help with my pain today. For my daily comfort, I rely heavily on the Psalms. David, one of the writers of the Psalms, struggled with pain, sickness, depression, etc. The raw emotion he writes with speaks volumes as I often feel the same way. But despite the despair that David was feeling, he never failed to also speak of the hope he had in God.

One of my favorite Psalms is chapter 102. It's not clear who the author of Psalms 102 was, but some people believe it was written by Daniel or one of the other prophets from that time while others believe David wrote it. No matter who the author was, it demonstrates how one can call out to God in great despair and anguish, yet hang on to their hope in Christ. In verses 1-2 of the Psalm, the author asks God to hear his prayer. The following verses, 3-7, describe his physical pain, insomnia, fatigue, loneliness, etc. Verses 8-11 talk about how the author feels deserted by everyone around him, including God and is completely alone. But then, he changes direction in verse 12 and begins to expound upon the power and majesty of God. Despite his pain, he knows that God is still in control.

Verse 18 really stands out to me. It reads: "Let this be recorded for a generation to come, so that a people yet to be created may praise the Lord."

What an amazing statement! The writer of Psalm 102 knew that his faith would someday encourage others who were also going through trials. He was talking about you and me. This Psalm was written for us.

The Psalmist goes on to pray to God that he may go on living. He also glorifies God and worships Him despite everything that he is going through.

In 2 Corinthians, Paul also speaks of comfort and describes how our trials give us the opportunity to be comforted by God and then to comfort others in the same way.

> Blessed be the God and Father of our Lord Jesus Christ, the Father of mercies and God of all comfort, who comforts us in all our tribulation, that we may be able to comfort those who are in any trouble, with the comfort with which we ourselves are comforted by God. 2 Corinthians 1:3-4

Let me ask you a question . . . are you more comforted by someone who has led a fairly easy life and hasn't had any big trials yet or by someone who knows and understands what you're going through because they've been there, too? In the same way that we can be comforted by Christ, knowing that He suffered here on earth just like us, we can also comfort someone else using our own experiences.

CAN I BE THANKFUL FOR MY CHRONIC ILLNESS?

I don't think I'll ever get to the point where I'm super-psyched that I have Ehlers Danlos Syndrome. Some days, I want to throw a tantrum worthy of a two-year-old or just ignore everything EDS related, but I can't. It's part of me, and it always will be. So, throwing a tantrum would be just a waste of my much-needed and often limited spoons.

Let's see what the Bible has to say about thankfulness.

> Rejoice always, pray without ceasing, give thanks in all circumstances; for this is the will of God in Christ Jesus for you.
> 1 Thessalonians 5:16-18

Did you catch that? "Give thanks in *all* circumstances" (emphasis mine). It doesn't say give thanks in good circumstances or give thanks in only the circumstances that you enjoy. God commands us to give thanks in all circumstances. That includes the bad ones. So how do you and I apply that Scripture to our medical conditions?

First of all, that doesn't mean that we have to be thankful for bad things. What it means is that we should be thankful in *spite* of bad things and be thankful for what they teach us. Am I thankful that my kids have EDS, too? Absolutely not. But I am thankful that they have the opportunity to learn all of the things in Chapter Nine because of their EDS. The same concept applies to me and my EDS.

A few months ago, I developed an exceptionally large ovarian cyst. The pain hit me just as I pulled up in the church parking lot for the Wednesday night Bible study. My husband was at work and I was on my own with the kids so I figured I would just push through the pain until the study was over and we got back home. That didn't happen. About ten minutes into the Bible study, I knew I was done. I stumbled down the stairs to ask my sister to bring my kids home after their kids' club and then staggered out to my van, stopping several times to sit in the middle of the parking lot because the pain was so intense that I couldn't stand up. When I got home (you're right . . . I definitely should not have been driving, but I was so focused on getting home that I wasn't thinking clearly), I curled up in bed in the fetal position, crying out from the acute pain. It was like being in labor except no one was offering me an epidural. The next day, the pain had barely let up, and so I asked my mom to drive me to the doctor. We spent the whole day at the clinic. Twice, we started the ninety-minute drive home, only to be called back for more tests. They finally determined that I had a 6.5-centimeter hemorrhagic ovarian cyst, but since it wasn't twisted, they sent me home with instructions to alternate Tylenol and ibuprofen.

Have you ever tried taking over-the-counter pain relievers while you were in labor? It's like expecting a screen door to keep the water out of a submarine. The next four weeks were some of the worst I've ever experienced. I had brief moments of relief, but much of the time, the pain I felt was still comparable to active labor. I spent a lot of time lying in bed while my sister took care of my kids for me. Finally, the pain started to let up, and I was able to resume a semi-normal routine.

Okay, we're all adults here who have kids so obviously we know about —*ahem*—bedroom activities, right? Obviously, with a cyst that painful, there was no way anything was happening in my bedroom during that time. But, that lack of physical intimacy opened up some conversations between my husband and me that actually made our marriage stronger. So while I wasn't thankful for the four weeks of excruciating pain, I was able to see that something good had come from it, and I was thankful for that.

Recently, a young woman from a nearby small town community was hit by a car while crossing the street and later died at the hospital. Her mother, who had already experienced significant loss in her life by being widowed twice, shared the sad news on Facebook. One would expect bitterness, anger, etc., but instead, she wrote a message of hope and salvation in Christ just one day after her daughter passed away. The young lady was able to be an organ donor and save other lives through her death. In addition to that, her story spread across social media, and her faith in life along with her family's unwavering faith through the pain of losing her touched many people for Christ. Even when dealing with overwhelming grief, her family was able to be thankful, not for her death, but for her life and for the way her life and death touched others. They truly have learned what those verses from 1 Thessalonians 5 mean in a practical sense.

So when you're wondering how you can possibly be thankful through your chronic illness, focus on the good that may have come out of it already or that may come out of it later. What has it taught you? How has it strengthened your relationship with God? Chapter Two is a good resource for helping you find some ways to be thankful.

There's one more thing I wanted to share with you before I end this chapter. A few weeks ago, I was having a really hard day. My joints were giving out on me, I was in tremendous pain, and I could barely stand up because of the intense fatigue. The three older kids were at school, so it was just Davy and me. Davy is four but struggles to communicate thanks to Childhood Apraxia of Speech. He was helping me in the kitchen, and I was getting very frustrated because I couldn't pick anything up without dropping it. Our conversation is below with translations for Davy.

Me: Davy, I think I need a new body. Mine isn't working right.

Davy: No, mom! Ee-us!

Me: Jesus? What about Him?

Davy: No oo (No new). Ee-us or bo-ee (Jesus your body).

Me: Jesus made my body?

Davy: Yes! Ee-us or bo-ee oo! (Jesus your body good)

Out of the mouths of babes, right? No matter how much pain I'm in, no matter how disabled I become, I can know that Jesus made my body, and He made it good.

CHAPTER ONE WRAP-UP

- It isn't fair that you have a chronic illness, but neither is life.
- There are only two types of anger: righteous anger and sinful anger. Being angry with God is sinful anger.
- God isn't punishing you. Your chronic illness is a direct result of living in a sinful, broken world.
- God does have a purpose for your illness. It may be to help you learn to rely on God and grow closer to Him or it may be so that you can be an encouragement to someone else. You may never know the purpose, but you can rest assured that there is one.
- You can find comfort in God to get you through each day. The Psalms are a great place to start.
- You may not be able to be thankful for your chronic illness, but you can be thankful for what it's taught you.

CHAPTER TWO

WHAT YOU CAN LEARN FROM YOUR CHRONIC ILLNESS

NOT ONLY CAN HAVING A chronic illness teach your kids some great life lessons, which we'll discuss in part two, but it can also do the same for you. Without my EDS, I think I would be a very different person and not necessarily in a good way. Let's go over a few of the things that being chronically ill can teach you and me.

HOW TO ACCEPT HELP

Because of my Ehlers Danlos Syndrome, I have had to learn to lean on others for support. I want to be independent and handle things on my own, both physically and emotionally, but that's just not possible. Learning to ask for and accept help is something I'm still working on, and while I don't think I'll ever be there one hundred percent, I'm doing better now that I know and can remind myself why it's important.

As women and moms, we have been conditioned to believe that we should be taking care of everything on our own. We're told that we are supposed to be that Pinterest mom who does educational activities with her kids every day while keeping her house spotless and maintaining a full-time job. Many of us are trying to model ourselves after the Proverbs 31 woman, but guess what?

She had help.

She didn't take care of her family and her home while working to earn money by herself. She had help.

> She also rises while it is yet night, And provides food for her household, and a portion for her maidservants. Proverbs 31:15 NKJV

Did you catch that? She had servants! So, if you truly want to be a Proverbs 31 woman, I think it's fair to say that it's okay to have help.

Here is the best part about accepting help from someone . . . it gives you the chance to bless them. Think about it . . . when you are able to offer some assistance to someone or be their shoulder to cry on, how does it make you feel? Important? Needed? Fulfilled? By allowing someone else to help you, you're giving them the opportunity to have those same blessings.

In God's Word, we are commanded to humble ourselves before the Lord. Showing the humility necessary to ask for and accept help is biblical.

> Humble yourselves before the Lord, and he will exalt you. James 4:10

WHO YOUR REAL FRIENDS ARE

Nothing shows the true colors of your friends like going through something hard. You'll have some friends who will stick with you through thick and thin. They're the ones who will show up at your door when you've had a rough couple of days (or weeks, or months) with a chick flick and some dark chocolate. They'll text you to see how you're doing and ask how your latest doctor's appointment went. Hang onto those friends. They're absolutely priceless.

But then there will be others who will seem to disappear into thin air after you've been diagnosed. Suddenly, they're not available to go get coffee with you or they don't answer your text messages. When they do talk to you, they'll question the validity of your condition, give you tons of advice on how to cure it (essential oils, kale, positive thinking!), or refuse to talk about it all. They might get angry with you when you aren't able to do the activities with them that you used to do. When you mention that you dislocated your hip just by standing up, they'll suddenly come up with a story about an even worse injury that they experienced, like it's some kind of competition.

That's okay. Even if it's hard, let them go, but keep them in your prayers. Maybe they'll come back later and maybe they won't. If they don't, then they probably weren't your true friend to begin with.

With that being said, remember that most people, even your true friends, *won't get it*. They can try to understand what it's like living with a chronic illness, but unless they have one as well, there's no way they can truly get it. What's important is that they care.

To have a good friend, you need to *be* a good friend. Here are a few tips on how to do that:

- Talk about stuff other than your condition. Don't let it consume you.
- Be interested in what's going on in your friend's life
- Try to find activities that you can both enjoy.
- Be honest about what you're going through.
- Be happy for your friend even when they're doing things that you're not able to do.

HOW IMPORTANT IT IS TO FIND YOUR JOY

I think this is one of the most essential parts of learning to live with a chronic illness. When your life is a constant battle with pain, fatigue, and being sick, it's easy to lose sight of the joy in your life. But without joy, you can easily slip into depression and hopelessness.

You may not be able to control your illness or disability, but you can control how you respond to it. You can choose to respond with bitterness and anger, or you can choose to respond with joy while focusing your eyes on God. There will be some days when you need to cry, scream, or be angry and that's normal. **Just don't stay there.** Let yourself be sad for a few minutes, then get back up and keep moving forward.

Sarah Buntain, a mom of two who lives with Epstein Barr, Psoriasis, Psoriatic Arthritis, and fibromyalgia says that her illnesses have taught her "to look for that one special moment that happens each day." Be purposeful about finding moments or little things that bring you joy. Write them down in a notebook and read them over when you're having a rough day.

HOW STRONG YOU TRULY ARE

In the last four years or so, my Ehlers Danlos Syndrome has gotten much worse, to the point where I am no longer functioning like I used to. I now own a walker, a cane, and a handicapped placard for my minivan, and I've had to relegate certain household chores to others because I am not physically capable of doing them. My kids are used to hearing "Mommy needs to rest" or "Mommy has 'owies' right now."

In addition to that, when my youngest son Davy was born in 2014, he had significant issues eating and by the time he was two months old, I was signing the consent form for his G-Tube surgery while the nurse stood nearby and assured me that my precious baby would be in good hands while he was under anesthesia having surgery performed on him. Even after getting his feeding tube, Davy continued to scream nonstop, had constant respiratory issues, threw up and choked multiple times a day, and spent a good amount of his time in the hospital or at doctors' appointments. It was incredibly hard, both physically and emotionally. To this day, if something reminds me of that time, I feel physically sick.

If someone had told me ten years ago what was going to happen with my health and Davy's, I would have fallen apart because there was no way I ever thought I was strong enough to handle it. I used to read blogs written by parents of kids with medical issues and was amazed at their strength, convinced that I could never do what they do, day in and day out. I followed people on social media who dealt with what seemed like insurmountable health problems that scared me just to read about them and thanked God that I didn't have to walk in their shoes until one day, I did. I didn't know how strong I truly was until I had no other choice.

I hated it when people would tell me "I don't know how you do it" or tell me how strong I was when Davy was an infant and struggling so hard. I didn't feel strong. I felt like I was falling apart. I would often push his stroller out of the clinic after a long day of appointments and having to hold my baby down for more painful tests, buckle him into his car seat, sit in the front seat of my van, and break down sobbing. I would scream silently at God, asking Him how He could do this to an innocent little baby and begging Him to heal my son. When people would tell me that they didn't know how I did it, all I could think was that I didn't know either. But he was my baby and as his mother, there was no way I could *not* do it. I had no choice. Any loving parent would do the same. As for my own health, I've learned how to take it one day at a time and just deal with that day's issues before getting up the next day and doing it all over again.

Even though I do not feel strong, I know I am. I can make it through the days when I can barely get out of bed. I can survive another round of depressing doctors' appointments. I can be the person my kids lean on when their pain is too much. By the grace of God and *only* by the grace of God, I am strong, and the fact that you're still breathing means that you are, too.

HOW TO PRACTICE SELF-CARE

It's easy to put yourself on the back burner. As parents, we're especially guilty of doing this. However, when you're dealing with a chronic illness, it's critical to take care of yourself. Self-care is not selfish. Self-care is how you take care of your family.

I once saw an illustration of a coffee cup that read, "You can't pour from an empty cup." How true that is! If your cup is empty and you have nothing left, you can't fill someone else's.

When you have a chronic illness, you have no choice but to slow down and take care of yourself sometimes. I know that if I don't stop and rest throughout the day and occasionally spend a day doing pretty much nothing, I *will* hit a brick wall and crash hard. I'll be trucking along thinking how awesome it is that I can do all the things and then, BAM! I'm down. Once that happens, I'm physically incapable of taking care of my family at all. I may have to miss events or reschedule long-awaited for appointments with specialists. It's crucial that I take care of myself and know when to rest so that doesn't happen.

Part of practicing self-care is accepting that you will have good days and bad days. Sometimes, you'll feel like you can take on the world, but other days, you can barely lift one foot in front of the other. Days like those tend to be extra depressing if you haven't prepared yourself for them. Accepting that reality can help you handle the emotional rollercoaster.

HOW TO HAVE EMPATHY AND COMPASSION FOR OTHERS

Let's face it. It's hard to have empathy for someone else unless you've walked in their shoes. But having a chronic illness means that although you may not know exactly what someone is dealing with, you're going through some rough circumstances, too. That can give you a better sense of empathy for the other person. Be careful not to compare your experiences though. What may seem like a small problem to you measured against what you deal with every day can be a mountain for that other person. For instance, when I had my first baby, I thought that was *so* hard. Other than asthma, she was pretty healthy and for the most part, so was I at the time. Fast forward to my current situation. I now have four kids who are all affected by Ehlers Danlos Syndrome to varying degrees, one severely, and my health has seriously declined. We have an average of ten medical appointments a month between the five of us and the clinic is a three-hour round trip from our home. **This is hard.** But that doesn't invalidate how difficult it was with just one mostly healthy child. **That was hard, too.** The same goes for other people. Sure it's tricky to have compassion when they're complaining about a sprained ankle while you're dealing with severe, chronic, disabling pain, but put yourself in their shoes (not literally because obviously their shoes are not supportive enough) and realize that just because your struggles are different, that doesn't make them any easier to deal with. You can use your experience to find empathy and compassion towards others.

HOW TO BE ORGANIZED

Okay, I'll be honest. I haven't mastered this one yet, but I've definitely refined my techniques since my health started tanking. After Davy was born, I designed a chart to fill out each day so I could track his current symptoms, medications, and issues. I had to learn how to juggle the needs of my three older kids with Davy's many medical needs and appointments. During that time, my oldest daughter Katie began to struggle more with her asthma, and my second child Nate developed asthma that needed daily treatment as well. I also have a long list of medications and so between the four of us, the pharmacist learned quickly to pull out the big bag when he saw me coming so I could lug all our medications home. It didn't take me long to realize that I needed a good system and so, I took the suggestion of a dear friend and set up a "medicine tote" (we use purse organizers which you can find on Amazon) for each person in our family with all of their medications in them. I also turned an entire cupboard in my kitchen into the medicine cabinet where I organized the meds by usage (pain meds, allergy meds, tummy meds, etc) and person. I had to get organized, or I would have drowned.

When Davy was around two, I designed a printable medical binder for each of us to use (it's available on my website at www.sunshineandspoons.com)

because there was no way to keep track of everything otherwise. Necessity forced me to become more organized.

For those of us with a chronic illness, being organized can make a difference in our health. It can mean that you walk into a doctor's appointment prepared with notes about your symptoms so that you can get the help you need, and it can also mean that you actually show up for your appointments instead of forgetting until the doctor's office calls to find out where you are. Being organized can relieve stress and make our lives a little easier.

HOW TO TRUST GOD IN THE HARD TIMES

It's easy to trust God when life is smooth sailing and everything's hunky-dory, but as soon as rough times hit, our faith can waver. It may feel like your prayers are hitting the ceiling and God doesn't care about you anymore since He's not healing you, but that couldn't be further from the truth. Focus on the big picture. Could God be trying to strengthen your walk with Him or allowing you to go through something that can give you the opportunity to encourage someone else?

> Blessed be the God and Father of our Lord Jesus Christ, the Father of mercies and God of all comfort, who comforts us in all our affliction, so that we may be able to comfort those who are in any affliction, with the comfort with which we ourselves are comforted by God. 2 Corinthians 1:3-4

Even the Apostle Paul went through difficulties that he asked God to take away from him, but God said no because He had a greater purpose for Paul's suffering.

> Three times I pleaded with the Lord about this, that it should leave me. But he said to me, "My grace is sufficient for you, for my power is made perfect in weakness." Therefore I will boast all the more gladly of my weaknesses, so that the power of Christ may rest upon me. For the sake of Christ, then, I am content with

weaknesses, insults, hardships, persecutions, and calamities. For when I am weak, then I am strong. 2 Corinthians 12:8-10

Instead of focusing on "why is God doing this to me," focus on God's love and purpose for your life.

CHAPTER TWO WRAP-UP

Here's what you can learn from having a chronic illness:
- How to accept help
- Who your real friends are
- How important it is to find your joy
- How strong you truly are
- How to practice self-care
- How to have empathy and compassion for others
- How to be organized
- How to trust God when it's hard

CHAPTER THREE

DOES GOD GIVE YOU MORE THAN YOU CAN HANDLE?

I STOOD IN THE PRODUCE aisle of the grocery store making small talk with an acquaintance I hadn't seen in a while. She knew that my kids and I had health problems and was kind enough to ask me how things were going. I gave a brief, fairly watered-down version of what was going on and she reached over to give me a hug as I finished talking. "God will never give you more than you can handle," she assured me. As she walked away, I felt crushed under the weight of everything. Those well-meaning words "God will never give you more than you can handle," had been repeated to me by many friends and family since Davy had been born. Every time I heard them, I wanted to stand up on a chair in the middle of the room and scream, "But I'm NOT handling it! Can't you see I'm falling apart?!"

There were many times that I got home from a long day of appointments and fell apart in the safety and privacy of my room after I put the kids to bed. "God, I can't do this. I don't know how to keep going. Please, God, please help me and heal my son," I pleaded. I felt like I was falling apart from the pressure of living with a chronic illness while trying to be a wife, mom, friend, employee, etc. No matter how well-intentioned the words were, every time someone told me that God would not give me more than I could handle, it felt like a kick in the gut. Instead of encouragement, I heard, "You're not good enough. You're a bad Christian. You don't have enough faith." All it did was make me angry with God because if it was true, that meant that He was *giving* me this situation because He thought I could handle it. Couldn't He see that I *couldn't*?

When he was still under a year old, Davy contracted a painful MRSA infection on his G-Tube site. I spent hours at the emergency room with him that day while the doctor determined what type of infection he had and what the best course of treatment would be. When we finally got home, I was exhausted, physically and emotionally, but it was time for his next tube feeding. I gingerly connected the extension tube to Davy's G-Tube, being careful not to move it too much so it wouldn't irritate his stoma which was angry and inflamed. Despite my best efforts, I bumped his G-Tube and he started screaming in pain. Within a few moments, we both had tears streaming down our faces as I tried to comfort my baby while slowly tubing the formula into his tummy. Thankfully, he fell asleep towards the end of the feeding. I left the extension tube connected so I wouldn't cause him more pain or wake him up and laid him in his crib. Then I crawled into my bed, and sobbed my heart out to God, begging Him to take away my baby's pain.

"I can't handle watching him get poked and prodded and dealing with so much pain!" I cried. "How am I supposed to do this?"

At that moment, I had a realization. Sometimes, God *does* allow us to go through more than we can handle. There was no doubt in my mind that I couldn't handle the stress and demands of a medically complex baby along with the then-unexplained pain and fatigue I was dealing with. **But God could.**

As I pondered that thought, another one hit me. God doesn't necessarily *give* us trials, but He *allows* us to go through them for our own growth and to help us draw closer to Him. Look at Job. God allowed Satan to test Job's faith by giving him more than what any of us could handle. He lost his livestock, his servants, his riches, his health, and even his children. But God did not send or give any of that to Job. Instead, He allowed Satan to do it.

Our pain and struggles are a direct result of living in a broken, sinful world. Now, that doesn't mean that your chronic illness was caused by you committing a sin at some point and it doesn't mean that it was caused by someone else's sin either. This world is imperfect, and our bodies are imperfect. Between sin in the world and imperfections, we will have struggles. Period. Everyone does at some point in their life and in different ways.

Was the weight of being in constant pain and extreme fatigue so severe that I couldn't even finish emptying my dishwasher more than I could handle? Yes. Was the weight of watching my baby suffer, not knowing his future, if he even had one, more than I could handle? Absolutely.

But God never promised us that we would have easy lives just because we believe in Him. In fact, He says just the opposite:

> I have said these things to you, that in Me you may have peace. In the world you will have tribulation. But take heart, I have overcome the world. John 16:33

You will experience trials that are more than you can handle, but they will never be more than what God can handle. And when you are down there in the valley being crushed under a landslide of pain, you have two choices. Will you stay there, angry, bitter, and blaming God? Or will you cry out to God and draw even closer to Him, letting Him pull away the rocks one by one that are burying you?

> Hear my cry, O God, listen to my prayer; from the end of the earth I call to you when my heart is faint. Lead me to the rock that is higher than I, for You have been my refuge, a strong tower against the enemy. Psalm 61:1-3

God wants to be your refuge, your strong point. But He can't unless you let Him. You have to call out to Him when you don't have the strength to keep going. No matter how tired you are and no matter how close you are to just giving up, God has the strength you need. He never gets tired, and He never gives up on you.

So where does the phrase "God will never give you more than you can handle" come from? It probably originated from 1 Corinthians 10:13 which says, "No temptation has overtaken you that is not common to man. God is faithful, and he will not let you be tempted beyond your ability, but with the temptation he will also provide the way of escape, that you may be able to endure it."

What Paul, the author of 1 Corinthians meant is that God will not give us more than we can handle *without His help*. That's a crucial piece of information missing from the overused consolation that is meant to encourage others. Without that understanding, telling someone that God will not give them more than they can handle can have the opposite effect of what is intended. Our struggles *will* be more than we can handle if we try to make it without leaning on God for support. Also, the verse refers to temptation, not suffering. We will suffer beyond what we can handle. Paul says in 1 Corinthians 15:10 (emphasis placed by me), *"But by the grace of God I am what I am, and His grace toward me was not in vain. On the contrary, I worked harder than any of them, though* **it was not I***, but the grace of God that is with me."*

So the next time someone tells you that God will never give you more than you can handle, try to see the good intentions behind their words and gently remind them that this is, in fact, more than you can handle, but with God's help you will get through it.

The hymn "My Hope is Built on Nothing Less" by Edward Mote is one of my favorites because it speaks about the faithfulness of God and how He always supports you, even when the world is falling apart.

> *My hope is built on nothing less*
> *Than Jesus' blood and righteousness;*
> *I dare not trust the sweetest frame,*
> *But wholly lean on Jesus' name.*
>
> *Refrain:*
> *On Christ, the solid Rock, I stand;*

All other ground is sinking sand,
All other ground is sinking sand.

When darkness veils His lovely face,
I rest on His unchanging grace;
In every high and stormy gale,
My anchor holds within the veil.

His oath, His covenant, His blood
Support me in the whelming flood;
When all around my soul gives way,
He then is all my hope and stay.

When He shall come with trumpet sound,
Oh, may I then in Him be found;
Dressed in His righteousness alone,
Faultless to stand before the throne.

CHAPTER THREE WRAP-UP

- You will go through more than you can handle, but God can handle it if you let Him.
- People mean well, but their words can hurt. Look for the motive behind their words to see their true message.

CHAPTER FOUR
COPING AS A SPOONIE

HAVING A TOOLBOX FULL OF coping techniques is essential when living with a chronic illness. Think of them as your survival tools. In this chapter, I'm going to share with you a collection of the tools I keep in mine.

JOIN SUPPORT GROUPS

Support groups have been a lifesaver for me. From answering questions I have about my EDS (is it normal for a knee to bend backward like this? FYI, the answer is no.) to being a safe place for me to vent about things that people who don't have a chronic illness can't understand, support groups are a true blessing. Although getting together with people in-person is the best, it's not always possible, thanks to schedules and health restrictions. But we have something today that people in our shoes just a generation ago didn't have: online support groups. It used to be that people were pretty much on their own to figure things out after a diagnosis, but we don't have to do that anymore. Facebook support groups can be an amazing resource, and I love that there's one out there for just about anything you can think of. My first experience with joining an online support group on Facebook was after Davy got his G-Tube. I felt completely lost and alone and was desperate to talk to other parents of 'tubies.' Despite having an awesome support system in my friends and family, none of them knew exactly what I was going through. A few weeks after his surgery, I was up at two a.m. rocking Davy because he screamed and turned blue if I laid him down. In an effort to stay awake, I grabbed my tablet and started browsing Facebook. It turned out that everyone on my friends list was sleeping at that time of night (who knew!) and it took me only about three minutes to scroll through my whole newsfeed. So, on a whim, I typed "feeding tube" into the search bar at the top of my feed and lo and behold, a huge list of pages, groups, and posts popped up. At the top of my search was a group for parents of little ones with feeding tubes that had thousands of members. *Thousands*. I had no idea there were that many other people out there walking a similar path.

I clicked on the group, then hit join and all of a sudden, I didn't feel so alone. I had found my tribe of people who got it, who knew what I was going through. If it were not for that group, I don't know if I would have made it through Davy's first year.

Since then, I've found Facebook groups for just about everything I'm dealing with. There are groups for EDS, groups for POTS, groups for Christians with chronic illnesses, groups for parents of kids with chronic illnesses, etc. I have even started several of my own, Ehlers Danlos Syndrome Zebras for people who have or know someone who has EDS and Spoonie Mommas for moms living with chronic illnesses.

TRACK PAIN AND FATIGUE LEVELS

Another tool for living with a chronic illness is to track your pain and fatigue levels each day. Tracking your pain and fatigue levels can help you notice patterns in your health and sometimes even allow you to anticipate the coming bad days a little better. This can also help you make some changes to your lifestyle that may alleviate some of your symptoms. You can track your symptoms in a basic notebook or go high tech with an app for your phone.

LAUGH

Studies have shown that laughter can actually relieve pain and depression. Just a few of laughter's benefits are increased endorphins, improved blood circulation, and decreased stress hormones. So laugh it up. Seriously (but not *seriously* seriously). Watch a comedy, make an album of funny memes on your phone that you can pull up whenever you need a laugh, read a funny comic strip, hang out with someone who makes you laugh, or do whatever works best for you. Just spend some time laughing.

FIND WAYS TO BLESS OTHERS

At times, living with a chronic illness can make you feel useless or worthless. You may feel like you cannot do anything for others or make a difference, but there are countless ways to bless others even when you're stuck in bed for days on end. Doing so is a great way to take your mind off your pain. You may not be able to volunteer at a homeless shelter or help your best friend move into their new home, but there are other things you can do that mean a lot and can bless someone. I'm unable to work for more than a few hours at a time, but I can go sit with my husband's grandma a few times a week. I can meet a friend for coffee or tea to give them a break from life. I can send someone a text or a card to let them know I'm thinking about and praying for them. I can give someone a (gentle!) hug. I can leave sticky notes with Bible verses and encouragement around for someone to find. I can compliment someone on their new haircut or their beautiful smile. There are *so* many ways to bless someone.

TREAT YOURSELF

It's okay to treat yourself every once in a while. It's not selfish; it's self-care. For me, when I'm having a rough day of appointments, I find a few minutes to stop by a coffee shop and splurge on a hazelnut chai tea latte. If I'm home, I try to find a few moments to sit down by myself and play solitaire on my phone. Sometimes, you just have to give yourself a little incentive to get through the day.

BEGIN COUNSELING

Counseling is an essential tool in my toolbox. It wasn't until I started Biblical counseling that I was able to begin to accept and deal with my reality. I balked at the idea for a long time even though my doctor urged me to start because I thought that since counseling wouldn't change my situation, there was no point. Once I did start counseling sessions with my pastor, I realized the value of it. I was right. It didn't change my situation, but it changed my perspective and my attitude and helped me focus on God. If you have a home church, I'd encourage you to ask your pastor about counseling. If he's not able to do it himself, he may know someone who is. Another option is to call the Focus on the Family Counseling Services and Referrals hotline at 855-771-HELP. They can give you referrals to Christian counselors in your area.

FIND A HOBBY

Having hobbies can help to distract you from your pain and fatigue and keep you busy when you're not able to do much else. I used to enjoy going for walks (ow), playing my fiddle and guitar (hurts my extra-bendy fingers, and I get dizzy while playing the fiddle which makes no sense to me, but whatever), and sewing clothes (hurts to lean over the fabric to cut it out). Now all of those things are hard for me to do because of my physical limitations. I still do them, but much less. So, I've learned to cultivate my other hobbies and pick up new ones to fill in the empty spaces left by my old ones. I've always loved writing, but not being able to do other things has made me focus on it more, which is kind of how I ended up writing this book. A few other suggestions are crocheting, photography, coloring, reading, drawing, knitting, graphic design, playing games, etc. If you're still looking for your hobby, try a few and see if any of them stand out to you.

EDUCATE OTHERS ABOUT YOUR CONDITION

Something that helps me cope with my chronic illness is educating others about it. I write about it on my blog, talk about it when people ask, wear my Ehlers Danlos Syndrome awareness bracelet, etc. I have been interviewed by a newspaper and two TV stations about EDS. I've been able to guide others toward finding answers for the health problems that have plagued them their whole lives. I've received tons of emails and messages thanking me for speaking out about EDS. Being able to help others has given me a purpose in my journey. Educating others about your condition can give you purpose as well. You don't even have to start a blog or be on TV. You can start small with your friends and family.

DON'T DWELL ON IT

While you're educating others, remember to not get lost in your illness. Dwelling on it and thinking about nothing but your condition can have a bad effect. Don't lose yourself. Your identity is not your illness. You are still you.

BE FLEXIBLE

Another of my coping tools is being flexible. Life throws you curveballs on a daily basis and having a chronic illness complicates things even more. There have been many times that I had a plan for how the day would go and then I hit a brick wall of pain and fatigue and was in bed for the rest of the day or I've had unexpected doctor appointments pop up. It happens. You have to be prepared for the fact that things can change at a moment's notice when you have a chronic illness and be ready to roll with it. If you don't have flexibility in your coping toolbox, those unexpected changes can really knock you down.

CULTIVATE A RELATIONSHIP WITH GOD

This is the biggest and most useful tool in my coping toolbox. My relationship with God is what keeps me going through the rough times and helps me to encourage others as well. As with any relationship, it takes work and commitment to help it grow. That means that I try to spend time studying my Bible each day and praying. I like to use the SOAK method of Bible study which stands for Scripture (the Bible verses or chapter for that day), Observation (my observations from the Scripture I read), Application (how the Scripture applies to me personally), and Kneel (okay, I don't actually kneel when I pray because I'm pretty sure I would never get back up again). I like to set the timer on my phone for five minutes and spend that time praying because I've found that I tend to try to rush through my prayer time otherwise.

I also cultivate my relationship with God by going to church and spending time with other believers. Hebrews 10:25 says, "not neglecting to meet together, as is the habit of some, but encouraging one another, and all the more as you see the Day drawing near." Spending the morning in church and then again on Wednesday night encourages me to continue my daily devotions and uplifts me. Sure, it's physically exhausting, especially since it includes getting four kids dressed and out the door on time, but it's so worth it. If you don't have a home church, I'd encourage you to start looking. Sometimes you may not be able to make it to church thanks to your chronic illness. Many churches livestream their services now via Facebook or YouTube which is a great option for when you just can't make it there in-person.

CHAPTER FOUR WRAP-UP

Coping tools for life as a Spoonie:
- Join support groups
- Track pain and fatigue levels
- Laugh
- Find ways to bless others
- Treat yourself
- Begin counseling
- Find a hobby
- Educate others about your condition
- Don't dwell on it
- Be flexible
- Cultivate a relationship with God

CHAPTER FIVE

THE FIVE STAGES OF GRIEF FOR SPOONIES

YOU'VE PROBABLY HEARD OF THE five stages of grief for when a loved one dies. The first stage is denial, then anger, bargaining, depression, and finally acceptance.

But it's not just the death of a loved one that causes us to grieve. Having a chronic illness comes with a certain amount of grieving as well as we grieve for the life we wanted and the life we thought we would have. Parents with special needs children go through this process, too, as they grieve the life they thought their child, and in extension, their whole family would have.

"This too shall pass" used to be my mantra. I could get through anything because it wasn't forever. But then my health started getting worse, and I found that phrase didn't really apply anymore because what I was going through *wasn't* passing. It wasn't going to get better and I had to grieve that loss.

When Davy was about six months old, I took him to the pediatrician for a check-up. True to form, he spent most of the appointment screaming. At one point, the doctor was asking me questions while I stood in the middle of the room and did my usual swaddle/bounce/sway move with Davy to try to calm him down. The doctor looked me in the eye and asked me how I was handling everything. I smiled brightly to keep from breaking out in sobs right then and there and replied that the only way I was hanging on was reminding myself that this would pass, and it wouldn't always be like this. At that point, it was the only way I was making it through each day as new issues arose with Davy's health and he continued to scream constantly, refuse to eat, and repeatedly get sick.

"You have to understand that it might always be this way," the doctor replied gently.

While I understood that he didn't want to give me false hope, his answer took my last shred of hope and sanity. None of Davy's doctors could figure out what was wrong with him, and I'd already been told that he may never be "normal." We weren't even sure if he was going to survive infancy at that point. But to hear a doctor tell me that the situation might never change was absolutely crushing. I held it together until I got back out in the van with Davy before falling apart and sobbing in the front seat, hunched over the steering wheel.

Thankfully, Davy's doctors were wrong. Not only did he survive infancy, but he's thriving now. And guess what? That particular situation did pass. He doesn't scream all the time now, he loves to eat, and he hardly ever gets sick. He's the happiest little boy I've ever seen, and he doesn't let his chronic pain and fatigue slow him down.

But not every story ends the same way. In a way, Davy's didn't either. His Ehlers Danlos Syndrome affects him rather severely, and he struggles a lot. As he gets older, it will more than likely continue to worsen. The same goes for me. I have a chronic illness and it's not going to go away. Some days may be better than others, but it's not going to pass so I can someday get back to normal. This *is* my normal now.

I went through a period of near-elation after being diagnosed with Ehlers Danlos Syndrome. Finding out that I wasn't a bigger wimp than anyone else out there and there was a reason for the way I felt was life-changing. Everything about my life finally made sense. But after a while, that high wore off, and I hit the first stage of grief like a brick wall.

The five stages of grief are presented like a ladder, but in reality, they're more of a circle or maybe a big scribble. You don't go through them once and then move on with your life. You'll circle back over and over again. This applies to someone who is grieving the loss of a loved one along with someone who is grieving the loss of the life they thought they would have. It's not linear. There are ups and downs. But on the whole, knowing the five stages of grief can help you identify the stage you're currently at and help you deal with what comes next.

In addition to being more circular than linear, the five stages of grief also do not have a timeline attached to each of the stages. Each person passes through them in their own time and in their own way. For some, it's a quick journey where they may skip over some of the stages, for others, they may get stuck in a certain stage for a while. As you deal with your grief, you'll have one of two paths to take with each step. Will you let it pull you down and destroy you or will you turn to God?

STAGE ONE: DENIAL

The first stage is denial. I spent many years in this stage, partly because everyone else around me denied that there was anything wrong with me at all. Doctors would run tests that would inevitably come back negative, I looked healthy and normal, and I was told that it was all in my head and I was just being a wimp. So for years, I kept telling myself that it was stress from school, then stress from my job and planning my wedding. After that, it was pregnancy, giving birth, recovering from childbirth and pregnancy, and adjusting to life with a baby. All four of my kids were born within six years so I figured that I would eventually feel better when I was done having babies. And then my last baby was born, and I started getting worse. Yet that could obviously be blamed on the stress of having a medically complex baby so I didn't worry too much about it at first. Besides, I was way too focused on Davy's care to think about my own health. And then, he got older and healthier, and I got older and less healthy. When he was two years old, he and I were both diagnosed with Ehlers Danlos Syndrome, followed by my three other children. I wasn't in denial anymore that something was wrong with me. I actually knew it now. I went through a period of elation because I was so excited to hear that everything I'd gone through hadn't been in my head and I wasn't crazy. Eventually, that high wore off though, and I crashed hard into the next stage of grief. I would intentionally skip my medications and push myself too hard because I was in denial and I thought that if I just pretended my EDS wasn't there, maybe it wouldn't be.

For many people with a chronic illness, the denial stage usually comes when they first receive their diagnosis. They are often in a state of shock and denial about their future with a chronic illness. It's not what they had planned for their lives so they may try to downplay it at first. This can be detrimental though because it often leads to not getting the appropriate treatment or taking care of themselves properly. They tell themselves that it's not that big of a deal and it will go away on its own.

HOW TO SURVIVE THE DENIAL STAGE

Talk about your diagnosis with someone else. Talk about how it makes you feel, what it means for your life, how the symptoms affect you. Find someone who will listen without judging or trying to "fix" your situation. Your pastor may be a good resource, either as someone who you can talk to or as someone who can recommend someone for you to talk to. They don't have to be a certified counselor or another professional, sometimes your best friend or your sister are the best options. A support group, either online or in-person, is also a great place to talk about your chronic illness and connect with others who also have it.

Research your condition. And by that, I don't mean look at the first page your search engine throws at you. Check the sources thoroughly online and talk to others with the same condition. This can make it more real, be that good or bad. The point is to get past the denial and to be honest with yourself.

STAGE TWO: ANGER

After denial, many become angry at the whole situation. That's a normal reaction to something that seems like a huge injustice. The anger can be very irrational and spill over to your friends and family but try not to let it do that. You're going to need them in your corner.

When I went through the anger stage, I was bitter and grumpy towards everyone, especially myself. I felt a lot of anger at my body for betraying me, anger at God for letting me be born with defective genes, anger at myself for not catching it sooner, anger at the many doctors I'd seen throughout my life who had written me off as a hypochondriac, etc. The whole situation seemed horribly unfair, and we humans are extremely focused on fairness, aren't we? I found myself lashing out about things that were not even connected to my chronic illness. Like I said, this stage can be very irrational.

HOW TO SURVIVE THE ANGER STAGE

Be honest with yourself and with God. Confess your anger to Him and ask for His forgiveness and help in letting go of it. Take the energy of your anger and channel it towards learning more about your condition and how you can deal with it. You can even channel that energy towards helping someone else.

STAGE THREE: BARGAINING

This is the stage where we often try to make bargains with God. It involves a lot of "if only" and "what if."

"God, if You heal me, I promise I'll use my health to bless others." "God, if You take this away, I'll start going to church again."

HOW TO SURVIVE THE BARGAINING STAGE

Instead of bargaining with God, cry out to Him as David did in the Psalms. Pour out your pain to Him. He cares, and He's listening even when it doesn't feel like it. Remember, Jesus also suffered immensely here on earth, and He truly understands our pain. God offers us hope when we're overcome with pain and grief. All we have to do is give Him our burden and let Him carry it.

> Casting all your anxieties on him, because he cares for you. 1 Peter 5:7

STAGE FOUR: DEPRESSION

This is one of the stages in which people often find themselves staying for a long time. Depression is common among chronic illness sufferers. Let's face it, it's depressing to be sick with no hope of ever getting better. On top of that, people with chronic illnesses often have vitamin deficiencies and hormonal imbalances which can also lead to depression. However, this particular form of depression is a natural response to grief and is a step towards acceptance and peace.

HOW TO SURVIVE THE DEPRESSION STAGE

While you're in this stage of grief, you'll need to seek your comfort from Christ. It may feel like God has abandoned you, but nothing could be further from the truth. Keep the lines of communication open with Him. Keep praying, keep reading your Bible. On some days, you'll have to force yourself to do so because it will be the last thing you want to do, but it will be worth it. God tells us that we can always come to Him when we need Him.

> Let us then with confidence draw near to the throne of grace, that we may receive mercy and find grace to help in time of need. Hebrews 4:16

We can also receive comfort from God when we're depressed and hurting. In 2 Corinthians, He says that through that comfort, we can also comfort others which is an awesome thought. Being able to use my pain to pass that comfort on to someone else who's struggling gives me purpose and peace.

> Blessed be the God and Father of our Lord Jesus Christ, the Father of mercies and God of all comfort, who comforts us in all our affliction, so that we may be able to comfort those who are in any affliction, with the comfort with which we ourselves are comforted by God. 2 Corinthians 1:3-4

Depression is hard. It's painful. And sometimes it can be dangerous. With a chronic illness, it's easy to slip into the thought that death is preferable to life with all of its pain. Honestly, an eternity free from pain and suffering that is spent with my Father in Heaven seems incredibly appealing. But only He gets to decide when that will happen. For now, my job is to be here growing closer to Him and showing His love to others.

I've struggled with depression and suicidal thoughts since I was a teenager. I've even attempted suicide twice, but the first time, I couldn't go through with it after writing a letter to my family and the second time, it flat out didn't work which I wholly attribute to God. If you're there in that dark place, I want to share a verse with you that someone recently shared with me. It absolutely blew me away.

> I shall not die, but live, and declare the works of the Lord. Psalm 118:17 NKJV

Did you catch that? **I will not die.** Instead, I will live and tell everyone what God has done for me. If that is not a purpose, then I do not know what is.

Before I finish this section, I want to make sure to emphasize that suicidal thoughts should never be taken lightly. If you're having any thoughts of wanting to hurt yourself or end your life, you need to talk to someone immediately. You're not in this alone, and you don't have to suffer alone. I've been there and I made it through, but I had to ask for help from other believers, including my pastor to get to where I am today. You can make it through this, too, when you cling to your hope in Christ.

STAGE FIVE: ACCEPTANCE

Acceptance doesn't mean you're resigned to your fate or that you've given up. It doesn't necessarily mean that you approve of or are happy about your chronic illness, either. It simply means that you've made peace with your reality and are living with it instead of constantly fighting against it. Doing so allows you to move forward with your life despite your condition. It's like when you forgive someone for something they did to you. Forgiveness frees you from your anger and bitterness, and so does acceptance of a fact that you can't change.

HOW TO SURVIVE THE ACCEPTANCE STAGE

In order to survive, you're going to need to accept your chronic illness and learn to live with it. It's like living with a hole in your wall that you can't fix. You don't like it, but you can't ignore it. Sometimes, you're going to be angry about the hole, but getting so mad about it that you punch another hole in the wall right next to it doesn't change the fact that it's there and only makes the situation worse. When you do feel yourself becoming angry, you'll need to remind yourself that it's just part of your life and focus on something else instead. The only thing you can do is accept its presence and learn to live with it. On some days, the weather will be nice and it won't matter that the hole in the wall is there, but on the days when it's twenty below zero or pouring rain with hurricane-force winds, you'll have to work to keep it plugged or covered to protect your home. With a chronic illness, you'll have low spoon or bad days when your main job will be just to get through the day in any way you can just as you would also have to get through a bad weather day with a hole in your wall.

Focusing on the whole picture can be a bad idea with a chronic illness. Let's face it, it's pretty depressing to think that your whole life is going to be like this with pain, fatigue, etc. So instead, focus on getting through one day at a time. You can make it through today. Worry about tomorrow when it gets here. Today is your goal. It's just one day. Alcoholics Anonymous has the right idea when it emphasizes that thought process to its participants. You can do anything for one day and then tomorrow you can do it again. Twenty-four hours. That's it. And if you're lucky, you'll spend some of that time sleeping. God even tells us in the Bible to focus on one day at a time.

> Therefore do not be anxious, saying, 'What shall we eat?' or 'What shall we drink?' or 'What shall we wear?' For the Gentiles seek after all these things, and your heavenly Father knows that you need them all. But seek first the kingdom of God and his righteousness, and all these things will be added to you. Therefore do not be anxious about tomorrow, for tomorrow will be anxious for itself. Sufficient for the day is its own trouble. Matthew 6:31-34

Part of accepting your chronic illness is letting go of the need for perfection and control. As moms, that's not easy. I tend to not trust others to do things right or get upset because my house is *never* clean enough. But I need to remember to give myself the same grace that Christ extends to me. What is important is that I'm doing the best I can with what I have, not that things are perfect. I don't expect perfection from my kids. What I care about is if they're doing their best and trying hard. So why don't I apply that same ideal to myself? Why do I put more pressure on myself than anyone else?

Just as I don't expect perfection from my kids, God doesn't expect perfection from me either. He is more concerned about what is going on in my heart rather than what my house looks like. When I hang onto control over how things are done, I am taking control away from God and that is not okay.

It's hard but try to hide the cringing as your kids miss entire sections of the floor when they mop, or when your husband decides to fold the laundry (the wrong way!) so you don't have to do it. It's okay if the towels aren't folded just the right way, and it's okay if the floor needs to be mopped again. Kids aren't going to learn if you don't let them do things and practice makes better (not perfect because there's no such thing!). Your husband is showing his love for you by taking care of things around the house. Look for the motive behind the situation and the lesson to be learned.

My need for perfection has stopped me from even trying sometimes. I used to think that if I couldn't do something perfectly and complete it right then and there, there was no point in even trying. Turns out that doesn't get you very far with housework or other projects. My energy and pain levels often don't let me finish a task or do a super good, deep clean job, so I've had to change my way of thinking. Now, when I have enough spoons to tackle something, big or small, I remind myself (sometimes over and over and over) that it doesn't have to be perfect. It just has to be better. Sometimes it means that all I do is vacuum one small section of the living room that really needed it, or just clean the sink in the bathroom, but not the counter, mirror, toilet, shower, or floor. A little bit of progress is still progress.

In addition to letting go of perfection, you also need to be prepared for unexpected changes. Obviously, this is necessary when you have kids because they can completely turn your plans for the day upside down in a minute. Chronic illness loves to throw a wrench into your plans just as much as kids do. Sometimes I wonder if the two are in cahoots with each other.

If you're prepared for the possibility that things can change on a dime, it helps make those transitions much easier.

WHAT TO DO WHEN GRIEF CIRCLES BACK AROUND?

Like I said earlier, grief is not a linear process. It's full of ups and downs, and just when you think you've gotten to the final stage of acceptance, something happens and knocks you back to the beginning. Sometimes it's something as small as having to stop for a quick rest so you can keep going or hitting a brick wall that crushes the rest of your spoons on impact. Having my whole day planned out to be productive and then having it derailed and ending up laying on the couch for the rest of the day drives me nuts. I don't like having my plans changed. Sometimes, chronic illness changes your life in a big way such as an unexpected complication that puts you in the hospital for a month, the addition of yet another diagnosis, or the loss of mobility. Stuff like that can really knock you down hard and push you back to the beginning of the grieving process. When that happens, don't stay there. You made it through once already which means that you have a one hundred percent success rate. With God's help, you'll get through it again.

CHAPTER FIVE WRAP-UP

- Denial: This stage is often spent in a state of shock and denial that there is anything wrong. Talk about your condition with someone or join a support group (either online or in-person) and research it thoroughly.
- Anger: This can include anger at others, yourself, or even God. It is often irrational. Use this time to be honest with yourself and God. Spend time in prayer and confess your anger to God.
- Bargaining: This is where you may try making bargains with God such as "God, if You take this away, I'll start going to church again." Instead of doing that, pour out your pain to Christ.
- Depression: This is a natural response to grief and a step towards acceptance and peace. Seek your comfort from Jesus and keep the lines of communication open with Him. If you have any suicidal thoughts or plans, tell someone immediately!
- Acceptance: This doesn't mean that you're happy with your chronic illness, but it does mean that you've learned to accept it. Focus on getting through just one day at a time.
- Grief is more circular than linear. Changes in your health or situation can easily push you back to the beginning of the process, but that's okay. You made it through once before, you can do it again.

CHAPTER SIX

WHAT TO DO WHEN THE GUILT HITS

GUILT. JUST SEEING THAT WORD makes you feel guilty, doesn't it? My particular brand of guilt includes things such as feeling guilty for:
- Working or resting instead of spending time with my kids.
- Not being able to keep the house cleaner because of a lack of spoons.
- Making sandwiches for supper for the third time in a week because I'm too exhausted to cook.
- Not being on top of everything all the time.
- Feeling like I'm not doing enough.
- Losing my patience and yelling at the kids.
- Forgetting to take pictures or videos at one of my kids' special events.
- Passing my awful genes onto my kids.
- Not being able to go outside and play with my kids (thanks heat intolerance and POTS!)
- Not being able to work more.

I even feel guilty for feeling guilty. My mom guilt is compounded by the fact that my body seems to be working against me (during the times when it works at all). Having chronic disorders such as Ehlers Danlos Syndrome and POTS comes with an extra heaping of guilt because, thanks to the world's emphasis on perfection and being productive, I often feel like I'm not good enough or worth anything. If we as moms don't measure up, the world is quick to jump on us and point out our failures.

I'm sure you've experienced a similar level of guilt because you're also a mom with a chronic illness. There's the guilt of possibly passing your chronic illness onto your child if it's genetic, the guilt of having to be the mom on the couch, the guilt of not being able to be the parent you want to be, etc.

What the whole guilt thing really boils down to is that I feel guilty for not measuring up to the world's standards. Guess what though? They don't matter. Not even a bit. Instead, I should be asking myself, "Do I measure up to God's standards?" That mom guilt and the guilt I feel because of my chronic illness is caused by taking my focus off what God says about me in the Bible. Let's take a look at just a few of those things.

God says that I am a child of God:

> See what kind of love the Father has given to us, that we should be called children of God; and so we are. The reason why the world does not know us is that it did not know him. 1 John 3:1

I am made in the image of God:

> So God created man in his own image, in the image of God he created him; male and female he created them. Genesis 1:27

I was created by God:

> For you formed my inward parts; you knitted me together in my mother's womb. Psalm 139:13

My body is a temple of the Holy Spirit:

> Or do you not know that your body is a temple of the Holy Spirit within you, whom you have from God? You are not your own . . . 1 Corinthians 6:19

God is focused on my heart rather than my physical body:

> But the LORD said to Samuel, "Do not look on his appearance or on the height of his stature, because I have rejected him. For the

LORD sees not as man sees: man looks on the outward appearance, but the LORD looks on the heart." 1 Samuel 16:7

God created me for a specific reason. I may not be able to do everything that everyone else can do but I don't need to feel guilty for that because God has created me (and you!) to do what He has planned for me. As long as I'm fulfilling my purpose in Christ, nothing else matters, especially the world's yardstick.

> For we are His workmanship, created in Christ Jesus for good works, which God prepared beforehand, that we should walk in them. Ephesians 2:10

None of us are perfect. None of us are doing a good enough job according to the world's standards. Those moms with the perfect hair that you see on social media with the beautifully decorated, sparkling clean houses, the adorable children who never seem to have messy faces, and the outings that always seem to go exactly as planned with lots of social media-worthy photo ops . . . you're just seeing the surface. Beneath that surface and behind those perfectly posed pictures is probably a mom who's stressed, shoves toys and dust bunnies out of the way of the camera lens and threatens/bribes her kids to smile nicely for the picture right after she's wiped their faces off with a baby wipe. What you see online is just one tiny piece of someone's life and probably not a fully accurate one at that.

However, not all guilt is bad. Yes, it's actually good to feel guilty sometimes! Some of those things we feel guilty over are because God is giving us a little nudge. Bad guilt is guilt that you impose on yourself because you don't feel like you're "good enough." Healthy guilt is guilt that lets you know that you need to change something in your life. Think of it as your conscience which was given to you by God to let you know when you're stepping away from Him.

Here are some questions to ask yourself to determine if it's bad or healthy whenever you feel guilt .

- Am I worried about what other people think about me?
- Am I doing something that goes against God's Word?

It's time to change your mindset. Instead of feeling guilty each day for what you're doing or not doing, focus your eyes on God. Choose instead to live each day, each moment for Him alone. Focus on the healthy guilt that encourages you to change to be more like Christ and stop focusing on how you don't measure up to what the world says you should be.

Are you ready to let go of the world's guilt and focus on God?

CHAPTER SIX WRAP-UP

- Guilt is often the result of being more focused on what the world thinks of us than what God thinks.
- We need to learn to tell the difference between bad guilt and healthy guilt.

CHAPTER SEVEN
HOW A CHRONIC ILLNESS AFFECTS YOUR SPOUSE

WHEN MY HUSBAND AND I got married at the ripe old ages of twenty-four and twenty-one respectively, we both said the traditional vows to each other, and we meant it, just like every other couple who says those vows at their wedding.

> *"For better or for worse,*
> *for richer or for poorer,*
> *in sickness and in health,*
> *'til death do us part."*

However, we didn't anticipate that we would actually experience any of the negative sides of those statements in our vows. At the time, we thought that "in sickness" was mostly referring to colds and maybe the flu here or there. That was tested right away on our honeymoon as I came down with a nasty cold on day two of our trip. I ended up sleeping the entire day in the hotel while my new husband killed time watching TV until I was able to drag myself out of bed long enough to go with him to get some cold medicine at a nearby pharmacy. We were young and in love and believed in the Beatles song, "Love Is All You Need." As much as I still love rocking out to that song, it couldn't be more wrong. To make a marriage successful, you're going to need a whole lot more than love. Love isn't enough when your vows are put to the test and things aren't so great, the finances are so tight you can hear your bank account crying, and your health goes downhill, never to come back up. You're going to need commitment on the days when you don't particularly like your spouse, patience when you have to pick the 487th pair of socks up from the floor *right next to the hamper,* and a strong relationship with God so that you can learn to rely on Him when your spouse can't hold you up.

My husband had a slight idea of what he was getting into when he married me. He knew that I had severe asthma and that it affected my daily life, restricting my activity levels. When I was seventeen, my health deteriorated so much that I had to quit my beloved job as a Personal Care Attendant or PCA for a sweet disabled teenage girl. Several years later, right before my wedding, I went to the doctor with the suspicion that I had Multiple Sclerosis just like my aunt. Since I was planning a wedding on short notice (we got engaged in April and married in September that same year and no, it was not a shotgun wedding) and working full-time at a busy bed and breakfast that saw a fair amount of drama among the employees and demanding guests, the doctor diagnosed me with . . . stress. Looking back now, I can clearly see that it was actually an EDS flare, probably and rather ironically brought on by stress, but we had no idea at the time. Despite lifelong evidence to the contrary, I always believed I would "get better" and was able to blame my health on whatever was going on in my life at that moment.

When I was finally diagnosed with Ehlers Danlos Syndrome, I kind of forgot that it would have an impact on my husband and my marriage as well. At first, I just assumed that he was falling in line with everything the diagnosis brought with it and that his main role now was to support me because *I* was the one living with it, not him. I kind of want to go back to that time and smack myself upside the head for being such a selfish idiot.

Here's what I've learned since then . . . *your chronic illness doesn't just affect you.* It also affects your husband on a very personal level. Being aware of that can make a big impact on your relationship and can be the difference between your marriage surviving or failing.

Let's go over some ways to make sure that your spouse doesn't get left behind on your journey of life with a chronic illness.

DON'T TAKE YOUR HUSBAND FOR GRANTED

Make sure he knows how much you appreciate everything he does, even the little things. He may be picking up a lot of extra tasks and duties that you are no longer able to do, and it's important that he knows how much that helps you. Tell him *thank you* often, write him little notes letting him know how much he means to you, and brag about him to your friends and family (make sure he hears you sometimes!) or on social media. If you have enough spoons, try to do things for him, too, when you're able such as making his coffee in the morning, plugging in the bathroom heater a few minutes before he heads in there to take a shower, or making his favorite food for supper. You don't have to make grand gestures to show him how much he means to you and how much you appreciate him. Often little things mean the most and can have the greatest impact.

MAKE SURE HE KNOWS THAT HE DOESN'T HAVE TO FIX IT

Men tend to want to fix things. So when they hear that you have a chronic illness, aka something that's not going to go away and has no fix, they may pull back and stick their heads in the sand. However, ignoring it doesn't help him at all, and it can make the whole situation worse for you as well. Sit down with him and let him know how hurtful it is for him to ignore your chronic illness. Let him know that it's okay that he can't fix it and that what you need most from him is his support. When you have conversations with him about your health and limitations, be clear with him upfront. Are you looking for some advice or do you just need him to listen and let you vent? Let him know what you need from him before you get started.

KEEP HIM IN THE LOOP

My husband once told me that he felt like he was in the dark when it came to my medical care and our kids' care. That made him feel like he wasn't a valuable member of the family. I felt terrible when he said that. My intention had been to spare him the nitty-gritty, sometimes boring details of our appointments and treatments so as not to put any added pressure on him. I also didn't want him to feel like he was my dumping ground for all the information. Once I knew that he preferred it when I let him know what was going on, I began to try giving him a quick update after each appointment.

Let your husband know that he's welcome at your doctors' appointments. If you have a shared calendar, be sure to write them down so he knows when one is coming up. If you have separate calendars or he doesn't use one at all (the horror!), give him a quick reminder. If he wasn't able to come along to your appointment, talk to him about it afterward so he's still in the loop. Sometimes, just a quick update is all that's needed so he doesn't feel like he's in the dark and has no idea what's going on with you. When you have a decision to make regarding your care, especially if it's a big one, talk to him about it first and let him weigh in with his opinion. What happens to you also affects him, and he has a right to know about it.

REMEMBER THAT HE GETS FRUSTRATED, TOO

I hate to break this to you, but it's not all about you. You may be the one with the chronic illness, but your husband is going to need support, too. Sometimes, he's going to be frustrated and upset. This isn't how you thought your life would turn out, and it's not how he thought his would either. Guys are notoriously bad at communicating their feelings so pay close attention to his signals and ask him direct questions about how he's coping. Listen to what he has to say and when I say listen, I don't just mean hear him. Let him talk without interrupting, correcting, or arguing with him.

BE HONEST AND OPEN

Just as it's not a good idea for your husband to bottle everything up, it's also a bad idea for you to do the same. I spent a good year of my marriage bitter, angry, and hurt at my husband for not supporting me the way I needed. Do you know what I forgot to do, though? I forgot to tell him how I felt.

Finally, I exploded and let everything out (probably not in the best way, of course), and he was surprised to hear that I felt that way. He'd been going off the assumption that since I hadn't said anything, I was fine. Once I explained what I needed from him and why, he did his best to step up. He even opened up about some stuff that he wasn't too happy about either which helped me realize that it's always two-sided. He needed to make some changes, and so did I. Once we opened up to each other, things improved significantly.

REALIZE THE CHRONIC ILLNESS *WILL* CHANGE YOUR MARRIAGE

When I was diagnosed with Ehlers Danlos Syndrome, I didn't think it would change much about my marriage. But it did. It was a lot like adding another child to the family except it was much less rewarding and fun. We had to make some changes and adjustments to allow it room to exist because it wasn't going anywhere. For a while, it was the elephant in the room that needed to be addressed, but we kept living our lives pretending it wasn't there.

Change is inevitable no matter what, and the sooner you accept that your marriage will be different once a chronic illness is involved, the sooner you can both work on that adjustment stage. Your roles change, your responsibilities change, maybe you have to cut down on your hours at work or are unable to work at all. There will more than likely be some trial and error before you figure things out and honestly, just as you do, you'll probably be thrown for a loop again. That's the way life is.

MARRIAGE COUNSELING

Statistics show that seventy-five percent of marriages that involve a chronic illness end in divorce. In order to avoid ending up in that percentage, you'll have to fight for your marriage and find tools for combating the stress and strain that a chronic illness places on a couple. Counseling is not a dirty word, and it doesn't mean you're in the throes of divorce, desperate for that one last chance to save your marriage. It's a maintenance measure and a way to learn how to communicate effectively, one of the most important parts of marriage.

But what if your husband isn't interested in or is embarrassed to go to marriage counseling? Then it's time to jump right in yourself. I put off starting counseling with my pastor for a long time because I didn't think it would have any impact on my marriage unless my husband was there, too. It turns out I was completely wrong. The eleven months of counseling I completed with my pastor changed my marriage and my life in ways I never thought it would even though my husband never made it to one session. It may be different for you. Who knows, maybe your husband will feel inclined to join you at one of your counseling sessions at some point or even start counseling on his own.

WHAT IF YOUR HUSBAND DOESN'T GET IT?

I spent most of my life being told by doctors and everyone else that my pain and fatigue were all in my head. Once I was diagnosed with EDS, I figured my troubles were over. Now that I had a name for what plagued me and could prove that it was a real disorder, everyone would believe me, right?

Wrong. It turns out that people will still doubt you and accuse you of faking it even if you have an official gold plated letter from your doctor confirming your diagnosis. The hardest thing is when your own husband doubts you. One little "are you sure you're not just doing it to get attention?" can completely pull the rug out from under you and send your world crashing down.

If your husband is struggling to understand your condition and its limitations, ask him to go to one of your medical appointments with you so he can hear it firsthand from the doctor instead of secondhand from you. It may be helpful to message or call the doctor ahead of time and explain why your husband will be at your next appointment with you so he or she can be prepared to explain the ins and outs of your illness to him.

You can also ask your husband to read articles about your condition and then discuss them with you, or you can bring him along to a support group meeting if you attend any.

If he still isn't on board, you may have to make your peace with that until he gets there. If that's the case, try to not overwhelm him with information and updates about your condition. Instead, give him small chunks at a time and don't push him too hard to talk about it until he's ready. Pray that God will soften his heart towards you and your situation.

BE SPECIFIC ABOUT YOUR NEEDS

Let's face it, men don't always take hints very well. Most of them actually prefer it when we're direct and to the point rather than trying to gently hint at what we want or need.

I'm definitely guilty of doing this. Instead of telling my husband that I need his help carrying the laundry basket upstairs from the laundry area in the basement, I'll lug it up myself, sighing loudly within earshot of him. Or I'll just hope that he notices me limping around, barely able to cross the kitchen and offer to finish unloading the dishwasher. Then, when I'm putting the last blue plastic bowl away in the kids' drawer and he's still oblivious, I'll explode and yell at him, as he sits there bewildered, wondering what he did wrong. One day, I was letting him know I was upset with him for not helping me since it was obvious that I was in pain when he stopped me in the middle of my carefully prepared speech.

"All you had to do was ask me if you wanted help," he said.

Oh. That was really all there was to it? The next time I needed my husband to do something for me, I skipped the almost imperceptible hints and got straight to the point.

"Can you carry this laundry basket into our room?"

Guess what? It worked! He carried the basket into our room and set it on our bed where I could easily take the clothes out without bending over. I said thank you, he said no problem, and we moved on with no arguing. Who knew it could be that easy?

BE KIND

This one is pretty important, but it's not easy. Honestly, on my high pain days, I'm not a very nice person. I'm also unkind to others when I'm in a bad mood because I'm angry about having EDS. I tend to snap at my husband for every little thing and sometimes nothing at all. But it's not fair to him for me to take my pain out on him, and it's not right for me to do so. To put it bluntly, it's a sin for which I need to ask forgiveness.

When you are struggling to not lash out, try to focus on the motive behind your husband's words. Is he asking you what's for supper because he wants you to slave away in the kitchen even though you're in pain or is he asking what's for supper because he just got home from work and he wants to know what's going on in his home? Is he asking you what's wrong when you seem upset because he's annoyed with you or because he genuinely wants to know? Give him the benefit of the doubt and be kind despite your pain.

HE IS ALSO GOING THROUGH THE STAGES OF GRIEF

You are not the only one mourning the loss of the life you thought you would have . . . your husband is, too. He may go through the five stages of grief (denial, anger, bargaining, depression, and acceptance) as he deals with his new reality which is being a caregiver for his wife. Give him grace as he journeys through his own cycle of grief, and remember that he may not do them in the same order or speed as you. You may be on your way to the fifth stage already while he is barely into the second, and then maybe he will skip the third stage completely while you're repeating the fourth stage. Everyone is different and that's okay. Support him in whichever stage he is currently.

DON'T FORGET ABOUT SEX

It's true. Men need physical intimacy to feel loved, and women need to feel loved to have physical intimacy. This doesn't mean your husband is some sex-crazed animal; it just means that God created men and women to be different and have different needs. I'm not going to go too deep into this subject, but it is something that you and your husband will need to communicate about as it's a very important part of marriage.

I've found that it's not enough to just assume that if sex happens, it happens and if it doesn't, oh well. I have to make it a priority. Sometimes that means not folding the laundry after the kids go to bed because I'm saving spoons for later *wink wink*. Sometimes, it means letting the kids watch TV first thing in the morning while we *ahem* sleep in because I know that if we wait until that night, my pain and fatigue levels will have me passed out in bed the minute the kids are asleep. We have to be purposeful about finding the time and making it happen. When I'm making physical intimacy a priority in my marriage, we're both happier.

However, sometimes, physical intimacy isn't possible at all thanks to your chronic illness. You can use those times to build intimacy and closeness in other areas of your marriage. Recently, thanks to an ovarian cyst I developed, sex was off the table (and out of the bed) for quite a while. Although the cyst was horribly painful (seriously, it felt like being in labor for a month straight, and no one even offered me an epidural), I was able to be thankful for the experience as it brought us closer together in other ways. As physical intimacy was not a possibility, we had some good conversations instead about some issues that we'd been having and ended up growing even stronger as a couple.

SUPPORT YOUR HUSBAND AS HE SUPPORTS YOU

Your husband is going through a lot, too, and he needs support. Without the proper support, he could experience caregiver burnout, and your marriage could end up in trouble. In order to prevent that, you're going to need to support and care for him just as he's supporting and caring for you. Let him know how much you love and appreciate him and be sure to keep the lines of communication open so you can pick up on any signals that he may be feeling a lot of pressure.

FIND CONNECTIONS

Most of the guys your husband talks to probably have wives that are fairly healthy so they may not get it. He may benefit from connecting with others who are in a similar situation. Maybe that's a friend whose wife was also just diagnosed with a chronic illness or maybe it's a support group that meets once a month. Maybe sharing an article with him about the unique challenges of a marriage that involves a chronic illness can help him feel less alone. Just talking to someone who's walking the same path can make a big difference.

GIVE HIM A BREAK

Realize that your husband can't be "on" 24/7. That's exhausting and not sustainable long-term. He's going to need breaks, and he's going to need to relax now and then. Encourage him to go spend some time with his friends or even just sit down and play video games for a while without interruptions. As a mom, we need breaks from our kids on a regular basis so we can preserve our sanity, and, not that I'm comparing you to a toddler who needs constant supervision, but he needs breaks from his responsibilities occasionally as well.

CONNECT AS A COUPLE

Take time to connect as a couple without it being all about your chronic illness or the kids. Find a babysitter and go on a date. Reminisce about when you first started dating or got married. Try to relax and just enjoy the time together as husband and wife. Bonus points if you're able to connect in the bedroom after your date.

MAKE SURE HE'S TAKING CARE OF HIMSELF

Make sure your husband is taking care of himself. He needs to eat properly, exercise regularly, get out of the house occasionally, take his vitamins, etc. If he's not taking care of himself, he can't take care of you either. You know how the instructions on an airplane are to put the oxygen mask on yourself before helping anyone else put theirs on? That applies to the rest of life, too. It's not selfish to take care of yourself because if you don't, you won't be able to take care of someone else. Remember, no one can pour from an empty cup.

SHARE THE LOVE

Spread the care around. Ask for help from friends and family whenever possible so the whole burden isn't on your husband. Look into what services you may qualify for such as housekeeping hours through a government program or a ride to doctor appointments that might relieve some of that burden as well. That way, your husband isn't doing it all and won't feel as much pressure.

WATCH FOR CAREGIVER BURNOUT

Watch your husband for signs of caregiver burnout. He may not even realize he's experiencing it until the pressure and stress has built up too much. The symptoms are actually pretty similar to the symptoms of depression. Irritability, loss of appetite, withdrawing from family and friends, feelings of hopelessness, etc. are all things to watch for. If you see any of those signs, talk to your husband and ask him what you can do to help alleviate some of the pressure he may be feeling. He may benefit from talking to a counselor or your pastor, too.

STAY COMMITTED TO EACH OTHER

It may seem like the kind thing to do, but don't give him a free pass out of the marriage just because you have a chronic illness and feel like a burden. If he's already having those thoughts in his mind, hearing you basically give him permission to leave can make things fall apart even faster. When you said your vows, you both made a promise to each other and to God that you were committed to your marriage "till death do you part." That is not something to be taken lightly. God isn't okay with us breaking that promise just because things get hard. Life *is* hard and the only way to get through it is to lean on Christ. Make God a prominent part of your marriage.

> And though a man might prevail against one who is alone, two will withstand him-a threefold cord is not quickly broken. Ecclesiastes 4:12

You and your husband are stronger together and even stronger yet if God is included in your marriage. When things get rough, that means it's time to draw even closer to God and each other instead of pulling away. Express your commitment to each other and to God. We can't choose our circumstances, but we can choose our reaction to them.

But what if your husband is not as receptive to all of that as you are? That means you're going to have to pick up his slack and pray twice as hard. As I said before, you can't choose your circumstances, but you can choose your reaction to them. That means you also can't choose his reaction to the rough times. All you can do is make sure that *you're* following God's will and Word and encourage your husband to do the same. At the end of the day, he has to make his own choices.

CHAPTER SEVEN WRAP-UP

- Don't take your husband for granted. Let him know how much you appreciate him and everything he does, big or small.
- Make sure he knows he doesn't have to fix you. That's not his job and that's okay. Let him know that you value his support and understanding.
- Keep him in the loop with your medical information and decisions that need to be made.
- Remember that this is frustrating for him, too. This probably isn't how either of you thought your lives would be.
- Be honest and open about your feelings and encourage him to do the same.

- Realize that your chronic illness will change your marriage. Things won't be the same, no matter how hard you try to keep them that way. Accept that and move forward.
- Utilize marriage counseling! It can be life-changing for your relationship. If your husband isn't interested, try counseling on your own.
- Let your husband know that more than anyone else, you need him in your corner. Try to help him understand your condition and its limitations. If he's just not getting it, give the situation over to God.
- Be specific about your needs. Don't drop hints or assume that he knows what you're thinking or need from him.
- Be kind to your husband, even on your high pain and fatigue days. Try not to take your pain out on him.
- Be aware that he may also go through the stages of grief as he mourns the loss of the life he thought the two of you would have together.
- Don't forget to make sex a priority! If it's not possible, focus on building intimacy and closeness in other areas of your marriage.
- Support your husband as he supports you.
- Help him make connections with others who are in a similar situation to help him feel like he's not alone.
- Make sure he gets breaks from his responsibilities when he needs them.
- Take time to connect as a couple.
- Make sure he's taking care of himself physically and mentally. No one can pour from an empty cup.
- Ask others for help as well so the whole burden doesn't fall on your husband.
- Watch for the signs of caregiver burnout and address them right away if you see them.
- Stay committed to each other. A chronic illness is not a reason to break your vows to each other and to God.

CHAPTER EIGHT

LIFE AS A SPOONIE DAD

IN CASE YOU HAVEN'T FIGURED it out yet, I'm a mom. As in, I'm not a dad. To write this chapter, I had to do a little research because obviously, I don't have any personal experience in being a dad with a chronic illness.

It turns out that if you search online for information about the challenges that dads face when they're living with a chronic illness, most of the websites that pop up are written for moms. The ones that aren't specifically about "momming" it with a chronic illness are focused on chronic illness from a general parenting perspective. When I clicked on the general parenting articles, most of them turned out to actually be written to moms, too. I'm in quite a few chronic illness support groups on Facebook, and the vast majority of the members in the groups are women. There is a large assortment of support groups for moms with chronic illnesses, but I wasn't able to find even one that was targeted to dads. My search for books written for dads with chronic illnesses on Amazon yielded exactly one picture book written for children with chronically ill dads.

I know there are dads out there who are living with chronic illnesses, though, so why isn't there any information or support for them?

There are several reasons why this may be the case. First of all, men are less likely to reach out for support through support groups, books, articles, etc. Secondly, women are more likely to talk about their struggles, including the ones they are going through with their chronic illness.

While most of the information in this book is written to moms, it's also applicable to dads living with chronic illnesses. However, I wanted to set aside a chapter to address the specific challenges that dads face. To do that, I interviewed several dads about their thoughts and experiences living with a chronic illness.

First up is Frank from Healthy Habits Reset. My interview with him is below.

Hannah: What chronic illnesses do you have and how do they affect you?

Frank: I have Celiac Disease, which is likely the cause of my Exocrine Pancreatic Insufficiency (EPI) and depression that I have suffered from since my teenage years and into adulthood. I have also suffered from very, very intense environmental allergies, asthma, and eczema. It doesn't have a tremendous effect on me anymore because I have put it in remission, thankfully! But not too long ago I suffered greatly from extreme exhaustion, some very prominent bathroom incidents, and the constant flares of my eczema, asthma, and/or allergies. Now, I just avoid gluten and make sure I eat an entirely organic diet, humanely raised meats, and avoid foods that I have sensitivities to (corn, dairy, a few others), and life is great!

Hannah: How many kids do you have and how old are they?

Frank: I have two children currently (would love more). A two-year-old daughter and eight-month-old son.

Hannah: What has living with a chronic illness taught you?

Frank: Chronic illness has taught me a number of things. The most valuable lessons have been becoming my own advocate, paying close attention to what goes in and on my body, and that God has a very unique way of showing us that He is present, and cares.

For instance, my wife also has an autoimmune disease, and we were diagnosed in the same month, around two years after we started dating! If that's not a match made in heaven, I don't know what is.

Hannah: What do you think your chronic illness has taught your children?

Frank: They are a little young still, but my oldest is starting to understand that our behaviors are different than other people's, even those that are close to us, like family. Since we cook ninety-nine percent of what we eat from scratch and make many of our own household cleaning and cosmetic products, we end up spending a lot of time at home. As a result, our family is together often, and we work as a unit instead of being separated like so many families exist nowadays. I think there is an old school vibe to how we approach life, and I'm excited that our children get to witness our closeness from a young age.

Hannah: What are some of the unique challenges you face as a dad with a chronic illness?

Frank: My autoimmune disease presents some challenges, but my approach to being a dad with a chronic illness also simplifies things. As I mentioned before, I spend a ton of time with my family, and I feel better now than I ever have. Both of these things come as a result of my lifestyle. My family time is abundant because I make sure I am home to help cook and clean. Since my wife also has an autoimmune disease, we share the burdens of maintaining a household. Plus, I feel so great because Celiac Disease has a very positive remission status—it's almost symptom-less with the right lifestyle.

The challenges come from any time I have to deviate from the "norm." So, vacations, for example, aren't as easy as just picking a spot and booking a hotel. I don't trust many restaurants now after some "glutening" incidents, so we have to pick a room that has a kitchen for us to make our own food, and is near a Whole Foods, or some other health foods store for the groceries.

I also don't get to go out very frequently with friends or coworkers due to the amount of time I spend at home to make sure we maintain our lifestyle that keeps us healthy. Plus, if I or the family do go out with other people, we usually just end up watching everyone else eat, which can be awkward for all parties. Similarly, I have offended relatives by turning down food (prepared especially for me) because it is not prepared correctly. Food is a *very* sensitive topic.

Abrupt travel for work can also be complicated, especially if I don't have access to safe food. And due to the nature of our lifestyle, we spend *a lot* of money on food and supplements instead of the latest gadgets or going out, which might be construed as challenging. But honestly, learning to let go of those material things has helped me to *love* the small and intimate moments that are often overlooked when you focus on moving fast and "living life to the fullest." I think my life is perfectly full.

Hannah: How do you think those challenges differ from what moms with chronic illnesses deal with?

Frank: That's a loaded question. Moms and dads have the same challenges in theory. But there are so many intricacies of being male or female that play into this scenario. I'm not even sure where to start, but I'll try to simplify.

I think moms are inherently more nurturing and the natural caretakers. So, a mom with a chronic illness has one arm tied behind her back. Her energy is likely depleted, but she still has to deal with whatever disease she has, raise a family, possibly work, and likely maintain the household (haven't met many men who help in this department well enough to take over for the mom). This means that she can get discouraged when she can't accomplish everything and has to work extra hard just to maintain normalcy. Since dads aren't as nurturing, moms might not get as much support as if the roles were reversed.

Whereas a dad with a chronic illness has a wife with instincts to approach things naturally —which in terms of chronic illness, is the way to go (while not being totally ignorant of western medicine of course). I feel like a dad with a chronic illness has more opportunities to relax versus a mom in a similar position. This is very general but based on my observations, not terribly far off. The bigger issue is that dads usually let their health fall to the wayside or fail to prioritize it over things that don't really matter. For instance, instead of changing his lifestyle or diet, a dad would rather take a pill that has numerous side-effects and eventually leads to more of the same. A dad isn't willing to make the same sacrifices as a mom, even if his family is begging him to.

Hannah: What are some ways you cope with your chronic illness?

Frank: The ways I cope with my illness are a *very* clean and self-prepared diet, a non-toxic lifestyle in terms of personal care products, cleaning products, etc., as much sleep as a parent of two young children can get, tailored supplementation including digestive enzymes, complete abstinence from gluten, of course, and a consistent, strong relationship with God. Without Him, I would surely be in the trenches of depression.

Hannah: Do you find it easy or hard to ask for or accept help? Why?

Frank: Personally, I have had to learn to ask for help. Simply put, I can be prideful or internalize my feelings when things get difficult (like most men), and I'm working to reduce that. We all need help of some kind, and I just need to continue to recognize that. In the past, I would hold any objections to food someone offered me because I didn't want to inconvenience or offend them. Now, I know that if I want to stay healthy, I have to ask them to help me by respecting that I can't risk eating their food. I just continue to learn how to accept these things and make sure I ask my wife for a break or some help when I need it.

Hannah: What kind of a support system do you have?

Frank: Probably the best one. I mean seriously, my wife (super-partner) has an autoimmune disease as well, and we approach our healing in an almost identical way. It works for us, and we have learned how to lean on each other easily. Plus, I have some pretty amazing in-laws that have learned how to cook for us, and always help us out if we need a small break from the grind.

Hannah: Are you a member of any support groups (online or in-person)? Why or why not?

Frank: I'm not in any support groups currently, nor did I ever use them. From my perspective, I never really went and searched for them because I had my wife to bounce ideas off of and to act as my support. However, several other men I know, who have chronic illnesses, do not use support groups either. I think part of it is a "man" thing. We feel like we have to do everything on our own or it makes us look weak or needy. And I don't even think it is a conscious thought! We have just been of a single mindset for so long that our actions are innate, so we ignore things like Facebook groups, blogs, or other communal means of help and struggle to maximize our health.

Hannah: What are some tips you have for the days when you have to parent from the couch or your bed?

Frank: Funny, I actually parented from the floor today. But whenever I am absolutely exhausted and can't bring myself to move, the best thing you can do with young ones is to bring them close to you and act as a jungle gym. It gives you time to rest (albeit not very restful) and allows a version of relaxation. If I had older children, I would engage in quiet conversation with them. Parenting doesn't have to be an obstacle. Let your children come up with the ideas and rope them in enough so you can keep up! The most important thing is to be together, as a family.

Hannah: Is there anything else you would like to add to this?

Frank: *Yes*. Dads with chronic illnesses need to take care of themselves just as much as they take care of their family. *Way* too often we intentionally draw the short end of the stick and do not give ourselves the proper nutrition, sleep, or support (whatever it may be). Instead, we put everyone else ahead of us. I don't think we even mean to.

The best part is moms do the same thing. Sometimes it is a part of the job. But we still can't lose sight of our health. If our children see us ignoring the critical components of our life, they will observe and repeat. Just look at the workaholic, fast-food-riddled, pharmaceutical-dependent, godless society we live in! This isn't a mystery; it is a result of pure disregard of all the things that actually matter.

Now, dads without chronic illness . . . there is a message for you, too! If your wife has a chronic illness, it's easy. Support her. If that means not eating bread or something else you love, take it for the team. Your wife is worth ten lifetimes of that stuff.

But finally, my message to everyone . . . I mentioned something about the direction of our society. We ALL need to understand that what we eat and drink, and the environment we live in, matters. We have ignored these things for long enough. So I urge you to become your own advocate, and stop *depending* on the opinions of others and to take your faith, family, and health into your own hands!

In addition to talking with Frank, I also had the opportunity to interview Sean from sobrien37.wixsite.com/seanobrien. His interview is below.

Hannah: What chronic illnesses do you have and how do they affect you?

Sean: I have Ehlers Danlos Syndrome, Dysautonomia, Raynaud's Syndrome, Mast Cell Activation Disorder, fibromyalgia, chronic fatigue syndrome, Epstein Barre, exercise intolerance, severe migraines, ankylosing spondylitis, unstable spine and unstable cervical, several bulged discs and disc herniations, dyslexia, eye issues, light sensitivity and sensitivity to the sun. A DNA test also showed the possibility of two other connective tissue disorders, Stickler Syndrome and Marshall's Syndrome.

Hannah: How many kids do you have and how old are they?

Sean: I have two daughters, ages 28 and 25, and one son, age 17. All three children also have Ehlers Danlos Syndrome.

Hannah: What has living with a chronic illness taught you?

Sean: Never judge a book by its cover. EDS is an invisible illness. People seem to think just because you look okay, that you're lying about the way you feel or that it's all in your head. Just because you're ill or disabled doesn't mean that you can't have fun. You need to appreciate the good things in life. The bad days teach you just how important the good days are. It's okay to say no, cancel, postpone, and reschedule when you're having a bad day. You find out who your true friends are, and they're the ones that don't disappear from your life. All of that applies at work, at home, with family, and unfortunately, even more with your church family.

I've had to learn that I am my best physician. It's sad how few in the medical field know about Ehlers Danlos Syndrome and even fewer will take the time to learn about it to help you. It's even more frustrating how many in the medical field pretend to know all about it, but as they talk you see how ignorant they are on the subject, and not just EDS but all the other medical conditions that can come with it.

I can't do the things I used to, and that's okay. I can find other things to do. My dad always said, "Don't let the things you can't do, stop you from doing the things you can do." I don't know if he is the author of that statement or where he read it, but it's a way of life for me. Being a musician, I used to be able to write a song and record it, playing and singing all the parts in just one day. Now it takes me months.

It's also taught me how important my wife and children are to me. They help and encourage me as I do them. I may not be as healthy or as active as I'd like to be, but there's always someone else that's worse off than me, and I can help to encourage them and help guide them with the knowledge I've gained through my health and spiritual journey.

Hannah: What do you think your chronic illness has taught your children?

Sean: It's taught them that life's not fair. Good and bad things happen to both good and bad people. We live in a world that is not forgiving and a world that expects the ill and disabled to do everything a normal and healthy person can do, plus more. 99.9% of the population has no time for my kids because of their EDS. So-called friends don't have the patience for their needs.

Hannah: What are some of the unique challenges you face as a dad with a chronic illness?

Sean: Being a father and husband with a physical disability has been hard. It has also been eye-opening and humbling. I've always been a hard-working, do-it-myself perfectionist. As my condition continues to progress and my abilities continue to fade, I've had to hire others to do the things I can no longer do. I've had to completely change my daily lifestyle.

Being a father and husband, I have always enjoyed having a family and being a provider and protector along with having my children to teach and spend time with. I also enjoy having a wife to be a rock for and encourage, raising our family together and looking forward to all of the plans and dreams we had to come true. Ehlers Danlos and all the other conditions that come with it have completely changed my fatherly roles. Something as simple as throwing a baseball in the backyard with my son isn't something I can do anymore as well as helping my daughter repair the brakes on her car or helping my other daughter remodel her kitchen. Spending a Saturday with my wife wine tasting or taking our vintage Corvette to a car show are all things I took for granted before and are things I can rarely do now.

Hannah: How do you think those challenges differ from what moms with chronic illnesses deal with?

Sean: I don't believe the challenges would be different for a mother and wife other than the specific task. Maybe instead of throwing a baseball with her son, it would be baking cookies with her daughter or maybe teaching her son how to dance. I believe all things would be painful or impossible to do no matter if you're the father or mother. Some mothers play baseball, just as some fathers sew dresses.

Hannah: How does your chronic illness affect your marriage?

Sean: EDS affects my marriage in many ways. My wife wants to go places and do things while I just want to stay home and rest. If I go, I end up hurting more which means I need to take more medications, which means I'll have side effects from the medications, and I will hurt for days after. She tries to be understanding, and I push and push myself to do as much as I can.

Daily household chores and things that arise with having and raising children can be very challenging as well. In our case, it's more challenging because my wife was involved in an accident and has physical disabilities, too, but we work as a family to tackle these challenges. On days where we are both having a difficult day, we may do nothing but rest. As a family, we eventually get the chores done.

There are also challenges in the bedroom as well, as you can imagine. Because of the constant pain and the side effects from medications the bedroom is *very, very* challenging.

Hannah: What are some ways you cope with your chronic illness?

Sean: I have several doctors I go to and many medications for the different health issues associated with Ehlers Danlos along with more medication for side effects of medications I need to take. I bought an adjustable bed with heat and massage, use a shower chair because of dizzy spells, wear a neck brace when sleeping, use heating pads daily for muscles and joints, and a Tens unit daily for neck and headaches. I also use BioFreeze and peel and stick heat patches and attend an EDS support group.

Being a musician all my life, I am blessed to have lots of instruments, gear, and a recording studio in our home. Writing, playing, recording, mixing, and producing music has been great therapy for me. However, it has become more and more difficult. In my search for a second form of therapy, something to continue to keep my brain active and working, and something I could do with my son, I have become a video gamer.

Before my father passed two years ago, he surprised me with an expensive recliner that fits my body perfectly. It has heat and massage, and I can adjust the back and feet separately. This chair is the *only* place I can be where there's no pressure on my joints and my head and neck are supported which for me means no headaches or migraines. So sitting in this chair and playing games has been a god-send. I also use this chair when I'm writing, recording, and mixing music as well as doing research on EDS and other subjects. Thank God for technology.

I also have a strong relationship with God and meditate on His Word.

Hannah: Do you find it easy or hard to ask for or accept help? Why?

Sean: Yes, because I'm a self-made, hard-working, do-it-myself perfectionist who was raised by parents that said, "You can do anything you set your mind to," and I was raised with a belief in God whose Word says, "You can do anything through Christ."

Hannah: What kind of a support system do you have?

Sean: I have a strong faith in God, a great wife and family that are always there for me and each other, a great EDS support group that is getting bigger and bigger, and good doctors who are understanding. My EDS group is an amazing support group that tries to meet once a month and also is involved in spreading awareness of Ehlers Danlos Syndrome and the other health conditions that can come with it. We were recently on our local news channel for Ehlers Danlos Awareness Month.

Hannah: How does your faith help as you live with your chronic illness?

Sean: I have always been very strong in my relationship with God. My wife and I were in leadership in our church and were the assistants to the lead pastors. We lead the young group together and took them to many youth events. I was the Worship Pastor and Worship Leader, and we were also on the deliverance team. While we were still serving in the church, my health started to decline, and we began going to doctors to find out why. At age forty, I was finally diagnosed with Ehlers Danlos Syndrome. I continued to serve in my leadership roles at church and to work my day job in construction, but little by little, my health worsened, and I gradually handed my positions over to others, eventually stepping down and taking an early retirement. After thirty years of working construction and being a musician semi-professionally, my body couldn't meet the demands I was putting on it.

Stepping down from all the positions at church was very difficult. I really enjoyed leading people in worshiping God, and it was very difficult to let that go. Now our church doesn't even exist. I hope it wasn't my illness that caused its end after I stepped down and retired. But God was strongly pulling us to move, so we did. The move has been great for my whole family. God has led us here, and He is continuing to lead us daily. We aren't being used in church right now, but God is using us to help others with EDS. We have our daily challenges but when you're walking in God's will, life is good no matter how messy it gets.

CHAPTER EIGHT WRAP-UP

Dads with chronic illness face many of the same challenges that moms do.
- It's important to take care of yourself.
- Faith plays a big role in coping with a chronic illness.
- Dads need a good support system just like moms.

PART TWO

PARENTING AS A SPOONIE

CHAPTER NINE
WHAT YOUR KIDS CAN LEARN FROM YOUR CHRONIC ILLNESS

THE OTHER NIGHT, I FOUND a note on my pillow from my oldest daughter, Katie. In it, she wrote that she wished I would spend more time doing things with her instead of just staying inside where it's air-conditioned and "sitting around all the time." While I'm glad that Katie knows she can tell me how she feels, her note broke my heart into a million little pieces. I do the best I can, but my body just won't let me be as active as I would like. The next day, I sat down with Katie to talk to her, and we made a list of things that we *can* do together, including some things I'm still able to do on my worst days. She felt a little better after that, but I was left with the nagging sensation of intense mom guilt.

It's not fair. Kids deserve to have a mom who can play with them and take them places for fun adventures. They deserve a mom who doesn't have to take naps just to be able to stay awake until bedtime. They deserve a mom who has enough energy to get through the day and who doesn't function like she has the flu all the time.

But guess what? Life isn't fair, perfect, or easy. It turns out my mom was right about that.

Despite how unfair it is for your kids to have a mom with a chronic illness, it can actually be a positive thing. No, really. There's so much that they can learn from the experience, and it can make them stronger and more resilient.

I'm going to go over just a few positives that I can think of off the top of my head, but I'm sure you can think of more.

EMPATHY AND COMPASSION

Let's start with empathy, which is not the same as sympathy. Sympathy is feeling sorry for someone else while empathy is being able to put yourself in their shoes. Kids who have a parent with a chronic illness are often tuned in to others' pain or suffering and can be more empathetic and understanding towards them.

My kids can usually tell when I'm not feeling well and will encourage me to sit down and take a break. Sure, sometimes they take advantage of my break to eat all the Easter candy that I thought I'd hidden from them, but often, they all pitch in to help out.

One February night, I was doing bedtime on my own because my husband was working late at the farm; I was so fatigued that I fell in the hallway and couldn't get back up. My then-nine-year-old daughter, Katie, brought me a pillow and my phone, and then took over bedtime without even being asked, getting her younger siblings into their pajamas and helping them brush their teeth. She then ushered them over to me along with their medicine caddies so I could help them with their nightly meds and instructed each one to give me a hug and kiss good night. By this time, I'd managed to get down the hallway and into my bed, so after Katie had tucked the younger kids in their beds, she came back to ask me if I needed anything. When I assured her that I was okay and just needed to rest, she hugged me good night and went to bed.

I felt *so* guilty that night because my child shouldn't have to take over parenting for me. Seriously, that's *my* job while her job is to be a kid. But the pride in her eyes when she hugged me good night stopped me dead in my tracks. It made her happy to be able to help me. So instead of focusing on the guilt of not being the mom I wanted to be, I focused on Katie's happiness and pride.

Things like this happen at my house all the time, on different levels and with different kids. Nate makes sure to ask me how I'm feeling at least once a day. Anna will notice that I'm not doing so great, tell me that I need a hug and then proceed to give me a gentle squeeze before skipping off to go play again. Davy will bring me his favorite toy to help me feel better or just snuggle up to me on the couch.

That level of empathy and compassion is rare in kids *and* adults. Yes, I have to fight off a lot of mom guilt when my kids have to help take care of me instead of the other way around, but I try to keep my eyes on what's most important . . . that they're learning compassion and empathy through this. They're also learning to be more like Jesus with a servant's heart focused on helping others. Essentially, the goal of parenting is to raise kids to be adults who will make this world a better place, and if my kids have greater compassion and empathy because of my chronic illness, than I have succeeded in that goal.

TEAMWORK AND RESPONSIBILITY

Thanks to my EDS, I can't physically do everything that needs to be done to keep the house clean, and so I have no choice but to rely on my kids to help. Yes, they should be helping anyway because it's good for kids to have chores and learn how to do things around the house, but not having the option to just do it myself means that I'm forced to allow the kids to do the job, even when it's not how I want it done. Believe me, there are *soooo* many times when my Type A personality just wants to step in and take over. I've had to work at letting go of my expectations and focus on the bigger picture.

Rather than telling my kids that they're doing something to help me out, I emphasize teamwork and family. We all work together to take care of our home *because we're a family*. We all help each other, especially when someone's not feeling well, *because we're a family*.

To give you an idea of chores that are appropriate for your kids' ages, I've put together a list. Keep in mind that this list is meant as a guideline, and you should decide chores based on your child's specific abilities. You can find a printable version of this list at www.sunshineandspoons.com.

2-3 YEARS OLD

- Pick up the toys and put them in a toybox
- Unload the silverware tray in the dishwasher (take the knives/sharp objects out first!)
- Dust
- Put their dirty clothes in the hamper

4-5 YEARS OLD

- Everything in the previous category
- Vacuum chairs and couch with a handheld vacuum
- Set the table
- Clear the table
- Wash the bathroom sink (with safe non-chemical cleaners)
- Fold the dish/hand towels and washcloths
- Match socks
- Put their clean clothes away
- Feed and water pets
- Help put away groceries
- Wash doorknobs

6-8 YEARS OLD

- Everything in the previous categories
- Sweep the floor
- Fold their laundry and put it away

- Clean the microwave
- Empty and load the dishwasher
- Make their bed
- Wash dishes by hand
- Pick up sticks in the yard
- Clean mirrors

9-12 YEARS OLD

- Everything in the previous categories
- Rake the leaves
- Take out the trash/recycling
- Cook simple meals
- Laundry
- Mop
- Vacuum
- Clean the toilets

13 YEARS OLD AND UP

- Everything in the previous categories
- Clean the shower/bathtub
- Clean out the fridge
- Mow the lawn
- Shovel snow
- Change their bedsheets
- Vacuum out the car

Children thrive and grow on responsibility. Sure, it can be scary at first. I mean, think of how you felt when you first started a new job. However, that responsibility gives kids a sense of pride and accomplishment along with a boost of confidence.

The whole teamwork idea applies to more than just cleaning the house. Giving kids a sense of teamwork strengthens their bonds with each other and teaches them to work with others towards a common goal. They learn to work together instead of just bossing people around. The benefits of learning teamwork as a child are life-long.

IT'S OKAY TO NEED HELP

I've had to learn how to swallow my pride and ask for help when I need it, which is not something that comes easy or naturally to me. By watching my example, my kids are also learning that it's okay to need help sometimes and that it's okay to ask for and accept help. My children all have the same chronic illness as I do, so this is a valuable tool for them and will be especially useful if/when their symptoms worsen. This skill already comes in handy when my kids are struggling with tasks, even small things such as buttoning a shirt or brushing their hair. It's a work in progress, but they're learning to try their best and then ask for help instead of getting frustrated when they can't do it on their own.

Our society has an "I can do it myself" mindset, but the truth is that God created us to need others for support. Raising kids who know that it's okay to ask for and accept help means that they will also be willing to step up when others are in need.

Another thing that kids can learn from being able to accept help from others is that doing so gives them the opportunity to bless someone else.

Think about it . . . how do you feel when you are able to help someone in some way? Tired probably, but also really happy. You might be proud of yourself, feel accomplished or fulfilled. The bottom line is that you can be a blessing to someone else *and yourself* when you serve others. Allowing someone to help you gives them that blessing and turning down their offer takes it away. That really puts it in a new light, doesn't it?

GOING WITH THE FLOW

I'm definitely a planner, not a fly-by-the-seat-of-your-pants girl. But I've had to learn that my plans need to be tentative. Just like I can't guarantee that the weather will cooperate for a picnic, I also can't guarantee that I will be up to a planned activity. I will often power through the pain and fatigue as much as I can and pay for it later, but sometimes, my body just won't let me do certain things. This means that plans get changed, rescheduled, and even canceled sometimes.

As hard as it can be to deal with changed plans as an adult, it's much harder on kids. I try not to inform my kids of any plans we have until right beforehand, but sometimes that's not possible or I get excited and share the news with them right away. My kids are learning that plans change, and they need to care more about a person than about an activity.

ACCEPTING DIFFERENCES

Kids are notorious for pointing out differences in people. Like the time three-year-old Katie was shopping with me at Hobby Lobby and saw an African American woman walk by. Her jaw dropped and stunned, she gasped, "Mommy, look at that girl. She's brown!!"

In case you can't tell, we live in a very small town without much diversity.

There was no way that woman didn't hear my preschooler's amazed little voice. Without missing a beat, I leaned down to her level and replied, "Yes, isn't she beautiful?" Then I showed her that although we are both "white," Katie's skin was a different shade than mine and explained that everybody's skin is different, and that's good because how boring would it be if we all looked the same?

Or there was the time when four-year-old Anna was shopping with me at Walmart and noticed an employee who appeared to have some form of achondroplasia or dwarfism. "Mommy, look at that tiny lady!! Is she actually a kid? Is she supposed to be working because I think she's too little?"

After I was done cringing at my child's loud voice and unintentionally rude words, I resurrected my little speech about how we're all different and people's heights can vary, but that's good because how boring would it be if we all looked the same?

I think you get my point. If there's a difference, kids will point it out, usually at a high decibel.

But the more our kids are exposed to differences and the more we normalize them, the less often things like that will happen.

Nate has several classmates in school with various disabilities. Side note: I love how so many schools are inclusive now. My mom told me that when she was a child, she never saw kids with disabilities, either at school or out in public. Back then, it was normal to hide them away in an institution and keep them out of society. Not cool. We may not be where we want to be in terms of inclusion, but we've definitely made great strides over the last few decades.

So, back to my point . . . Nate has several classmates with disabilities. And you know what? They're not "the kid in the wheelchair" or "the kid who talks and walks differently than me." They're Adam and Henry (*names have been changed*). They're his friends, and they're just like him. Adam loves tractors like Nate, and Henry is a goofy kid like Nate. That's how he sees them. That's a perspective he probably wouldn't have if he didn't get to attend school with them.

The same goes for having a mom with a chronic illness. Being around someone who's different in any way normalizes it for kids and teaches them that people who may not look, act, walk, talk, etc. like them, are still just regular people.

So, what about the differences you can't see? Unless I'm wearing a brace or am using my walker, I look like everyone else. I look like a healthy, normal adult, something that couldn't be further from the truth some days.

People in the chronic illness community are constantly fighting to make their invisible illnesses "seen." You've probably seen stories on Facebook of people who look fine on the outside using their much-needed handicap placard and then coming back outside to an angry note on the windshield berating them for using a parking spot that some passerby decided they don't need.

Having a parent with an invisible illness teaches kids to give grace and compassion to others because they never know what they're struggling with beneath the surface. We're raising a generation of people who understand that not all disabilities are visible. How awesome is that?!

HOW TO TRUST GOD IN THE HARD TIMES

Trusting God is easy when things are going well, but when your prayers seem to go unanswered and your life is turning upside down, it becomes significantly more difficult. When a child prays that God would heal his or her mom so she won't be sick anymore, but doesn't see any healing, they can start to doubt God. It's important that they know that God is still in control even though sometimes He says no to their requests and lets them go through hard times. Emphasize to your child that God can see a greater purpose for difficulties in their life that they can't see. I've found that it helps to draw a timeline on paper that represents their life to demonstrate that they can see only a little tiny section of it, which is the past and the present. Then I explain that God sees the whole timeline, from start to finish, and He knows how this trial will play out. Something good **can** come out of it. Maybe it will be a stronger faith in Him, maybe it will be the chance to help someone else going through something similar down the road. We don't know until He shows us and that's okay because that can help build our trust in God.

Let's go back over that list . . . kids who have parents with chronic illnesses often learn empathy, compassion, teamwork, responsibility, how to go with the flow, how to accept differences, how to trust God even when it's not easy, and that not all disabilities are visible. That's a pretty awesome human being right there if you ask me.

So while it doesn't seem fair to your kids that you have a chronic illness, and it stinks that they have to miss out on some things because of it, look at all the things it has taught them. Write them down and focus on that list when you don't feel like you're a good enough mom.

CHAPTER NINE WRAP-UP

Kids who have parents with chronic illnesses can learn:
- Empathy
- Compassion
- Teamwork
- Responsibility
- How to go with the flow
- How to accept differences
- That not all disabilities are visible

CHAPTER TEN

WHEN YOU AND YOUR CHILD(REN) ARE SPOONIES

WHEN DAVY AND I WERE diagnosed with Ehlers Danlos Syndrome, he had already been dealing with his health problems for two years, so it was a relief to have answers. I desperately wanted him to be healthy and pain-free, but I had already come to terms with the fact that he would always struggle. At the time, I suspected my two oldest children of having EDS as well but was hoping I was wrong. My daughter, Katie—then seven years old—had started complaining of pain in her legs, which was one of the first signs of my own EDS as a child although we didn't realize it at the time. And five-year-old Nate, well, there was no denying that he was hypermobile. He often seemed to be made of rubber and slept with his limbs twisted in such awkward looking positions that it looked like he had been dropped off a ten-story building. There were a few other signs as well, but ones that could still be written off as something else.

Later that summer, I took Katie, Nate, and Anna in to see our geneticist. It was a crazy appointment as I was alone with all four kids and the exams and questions took several hours. By the end of it, I was saddened, but not surprised when she diagnosed both Katie and Nate with Ehlers Danlos Syndrome as well. Anna was only three years old at the time and the geneticist was on the fence with her. She didn't complain of any pain and was the healthiest of all four of my children. She was hypermobile, but that's common for kids that age and so the geneticist told us to bring her back in a few years to recheck her if we still had any concerns. Around the time Anna turned five, she began to complain of fatigue and pain in her legs, and my heart sank. Her hypermobility could no longer be attributed to being so young and appeared to be getting even worse. Reluctantly, I scheduled a repeat appointment for her with the geneticist. That day, my fourth and final child was diagnosed with EDS, bringing the grand total for our family up to five people affected. I learned that I had a fifty percent chance of passing EDS on to each child I had. My geneticist labeled me an overachiever as I have a one hundred percent rate of passing my defective genes to my kids. Go me.

Ehlers Danlos Syndrome is a highly unpredictable condition that can change with no warning and affects each person differently, and so there is no telling what my children's future will hold. Both of my boys seem to be more severely affected than my daughters, but I take hope in the fact that often the increased testosterone during puberty can strengthen boys' muscles enough to diminish their pain and symptoms so their bodies will no longer be working so hard just to hold everything together. However, girls generally tend to worsen significantly in puberty due to increased laxity in their joints. Obviously, there is no comfort in that fact for me, especially as I experienced that firsthand when I hit puberty. All I can do is give my kids the tools they need to be able to cope with their EDS and live the best lives that they can.

It's hard enough living with a chronic illness yourself, but watching your child live with one as well is absolutely heartbreaking. No one wants their child to suffer.

Maybe your child inherited their chronic illness from you or maybe they have a different one completely. Either way, this is a tough situation. How do you cope with being a chronically ill parent with a child who is living with a chronic illness or special needs of their own?

BE AN EXAMPLE

First of all, no matter if you both have different conditions or the same one(s), your child is watching how you deal with your chronic illness to learn how they need to live with their chronic illness or special needs. If you are angry and bitter about your health, they probably will be, too. Just as we as moms need to model good body image for our daughters by not making disparaging comments about the way we look in front of them, we need to do the same thing for our kids with chronic illnesses or other special needs. Your body may not work the way it should, but if you constantly complain about it, your kids will do the same. If you don't take care of yourself and manage your spoons properly, they won't either. We must model self-care and pacing so our kids can learn it, too. You can't expect your child to stop and rest when they see you constantly pushing yourself harder than you should.

My kids are now eleven, nine, six, and five, and I've noticed that they are able to recognize when they need to stop and take a break. They're able to self-regulate both physically and emotionally. At least a few times a week, I'll notice that one of them is missing from the general chaos of our house and will find them snuggled up in their bed resting with their eyes closed or reading a book. When I ask what they're doing, their answers vary from "I needed some quiet" to "my body is tired and hurting so I decided to rest." Davy hasn't quite gotten to that point yet, but he will find a spot on the floor and lay down when he's tired or in pain until he's ready to get back up. Not to toot my own horn, but the kids do things like that because I've talked to them about self-care and demonstrated it.

FOCUS ON THE POSITIVE

Having a chronic illness can be scary for an adult, let alone a child. While you want to be sure not to ignore those worries and thoughts, at the same time, it's best not to dwell on them. Instead, help your child to focus on the positive side of things. Doing so gives them the tools they need for coping. If they're going to be living with their condition for the rest of their lives, it's essential that they learn how to cope with it now in a healthy way.

Read back over chapter two about what having a chronic illness can teach you. That's what your kids can gain from their chronic illness or special needs as well. Here's the list again in case you prefer a brief recap over reading the whole chapter again.

What your chronic illness can teach you (no matter if you're an adult or a child!):

- How to accept help
- Who your real friends are
- How important it is to find your joy
- How strong you truly are
- How to practice self-care
- How to have empathy and compassion for others
- How to be organized

WE'RE ALL DIFFERENT

From the color of our skin to our unique talents, everyone is different. Your child's chronic illness or special needs are no different. It's just another part of who they are. They can't change it any more than they can change the color of their eyes. Every so often, one of my kids comes to me upset because their Ehlers Danlos Syndrome makes them different which means that they can't do the same things as their friends. When that happens, we sit down and talk about how everyone has differences and struggles. We talk about their friends and how there are differences between them all, in looks, personality, and even medical issues. Also, everyone will have hard times in their life at some point. Some people just go through them earlier than others.

WHEN YOUR KID'S CONDITION COMES FROM YOU

While getting my blood drawn at the clinic one day, the lab technician was extra friendly and talkative, which was fine. I like that better than having someone who barely says a word and makes you feel more like a vein they can stick a needle into than an actual person. We were talking about how my kids and I all have Ehlers Danlos Syndrome when she asked me a question.

"Why would you even have children knowing you could pass such a horrible condition on to them?"

I was floored. I didn't see how that was any of her business, but it turns out that many people since then have also considered that their business and have thought it was okay to ask a similarly worded question.

Up until that day, I hadn't really thought much about how my kids inherited their EDS from me. The diagnosis was still so new that I was trying to wrap my head around it and figure out how to manage care for so many people. During the whole ninety-minute drive home, I kept going over and over the conversation. It took me about a week to finally formulate my thoughts about why it bothered me so much and why it made feel so guilty and horrible.

First of all, I didn't know I had Ehlers Danlos Syndrome until *after* my fourth and final baby was born. I knew I had health issues, but I figured it was just my problem and my three older kids were fairly healthy besides some asthma up until they were in kindergarten/first grade. So then, I had to ask myself, if I had known, would I still have had children? After mulling that over for a while, I came to the realization that I don't think it would have changed anything. As it was, none of my children were planned. The first one came several years before we had planned to start having kids and then after that, they kept coming despite us using a form of contraception. Baby #2, Nate, was very high needs as an infant and screamed almost nonstop. He had feeding difficulties as well and it was a very rough year for our family. After that, I was ready to be done having babies and was happy with the size of our family even though I'd always wanted a minimum of four kids up until that point. And then, I found out I was expecting Baby #3. I was dreading going through the baby stage again, but when she was born, she was the sweetest, easiest baby ever. I was thrilled. She was the perfect finish for our family after

Nate's difficult infancy. And then, when she was only seven months old, I took a pregnancy test on a whim, fully expecting it to be negative. It wasn't. I'll be honest . . . I spent the rest of the day crying and they weren't happy tears, as I tried to come to terms with this new change for our family and going through another rough pregnancy. And then Davy was born and started our family on a wild rollercoaster of a journey that led to all of us being diagnosed with EDS.

I grew up with undiagnosed Ehlers Danlos Syndrome. Despite all my struggles and being told repeatedly that it was all in my head, I don't regret my life. I'm glad I was born, and I'm glad I've lived it. I'm even thankful for the way my EDS has shaped my life and enriched it in some ways. Despite my health, I've enjoyed my life for the most part. Sure, there have been some moments where it wasn't so enjoyable, but I think that's normal for everyone. I hope my children grow up to also have the perspective that life is still worth living even when it's hard.

By saying that someone should not have children because those children could have a condition that makes them less than perfect in the world's eyes is saying that those children are not worthy of life. As I said before, we're all different. We all struggle. We all have strengths and weaknesses. Imagine a world where everyone is the same and there are no people with disabilities or special needs. Families and society, in general, would lose so much such as empathy, a sense of understanding for those different than you, etc. Just because someone is different than what society has labeled as normal does not mean their life is not worth living. Our greatest weaknesses can become the greatest blessings to us and others if we allow them.

DEPRESSION IN YOUR CHILD

Anyone living with a chronic illness is at high risk for depression. That includes children. They have to deal with some very grown-up emotions at an early age because of their illness. I had undiagnosed EDS as a child, but I did have a diagnosis of severe asthma. It was bad enough that I nearly died several times. At the age of six, I stopped breathing and was in a medically induced coma for five days. Despite having blocked the actual event out of my memory (which is something young children often do when they experience a traumatic event), I remember very distinctly being depressed after that and couldn't figure out why. When I was seven years old, I told my grandpa that I thought seven should be a good year because it rhymed with heaven (the logic of a child), but I just wasn't happy. When I was ten, I had another severe asthma attack that nearly killed me, and this time, I didn't block it out. After that, I started having panic attacks whenever I saw or heard an ambulance or smelled antiseptic/hospital smells. Every time I thought my panic attacks were getting "better," I would have another severe asthma attack and end up worse than before.

Unfortunately, I didn't get any help for my depression and PTSD when I was young and by the time I was in my upper teens, it had worsened significantly. I went through many years of depression, suicidal thoughts, and two attempts at suicide before finally getting help for it in my thirties. As a parent myself, I now watch my kids closely for any signs of depression, knowing that they are at high-risk thanks to their EDS.

Here's what you should watch for in your child. If they show any of these signs of being depressed, find someone such as a counselor, therapist, pastor, etc. for them to talk to.

- Mood swings
- Changes in sleeping and eating habits
- A slip in grades at school
- Fighting constantly with their family and/or friends or losing interest in spending time with them
- Making negative comments about themselves
- A sudden change in behavior such as tantrums or fear
- Looking unhappy, angry, or sad
- Losing interest in things that he or she used to love
- Talking about death and dying

GETTING ORGANIZED

Being organized when you have a chronic illness is important and even much more when your child also has a chronic illness or special needs. Brain fog can make it extremely difficult to remember what questions you have for your child's doctor or what was discussed at the appointment. It can lead to missed appointments and medication dosages. It's hard enough trying to keep track of your own medical information, let alone someone else's.

When it comes to doctor appointments and therapies, I try to schedule follow-ups right away while we're still at the clinic or request a reminder letter if the next appointment is too far away to schedule yet. I used to keep a paper planner in my purse but have switched to using the calendar on my phone to cut down on the weight of my purse. That also makes it easier to search for past and future appointments and I can sync it to my husband's phone, so he knows where we are that day. Since we live ninety minutes from our clinic, I try to schedule multiple appointments in one day to cut down on the number of days we have to spend at the clinic each week. With five people in one family who all have EDS as well as asthma, severe eczema, etc., we have an average of ten to fifteen appointments each month so cramming two to four appointments into one visit helps cut down on the number of days we're gone.

After yet another asthma attack put me in the hospital overnight a few years ago, I realized that I needed to not be the only person capable of caring for my kids' medical needs. At the time, Davy still had a feeding tube and although I had taught several family members how to tube feed him, I hadn't told anyone how to do his tube and skin-care routine to keep his stoma healthy and his eczema somewhat under control, the protocol for his lungs as he had frequent issues with them, how to determine how much to feed him, or how to tell when he was going to start choking and throw up. Despite being well taken care of while I was gone, it took several weeks to get Davy's stoma and eczema back to a healthy state again just from that one night of me not taking care of it. It definitely wasn't a good idea to be the only one who knew what to do for him. On top of that, no one else knew the dosing for Katie and Nate's asthma medication.

I realized that I needed to put together a care plan for my kids so that others could care for them properly if something were to happen to me again. I also decided to organize my kids' medications into a small bag for each of them where I could also keep a chart of the dosage and time each medication needed to be taken along with a copy of their care plan. Those bags sit on top of a dresser where the kids can reach them so that they can handle their medication on their own (I still supervise, though!).

I highly recommend setting up a care plan for your child. Even healthy moms can suddenly become ill or be in an accident and if you have a chronic illness, there's a much higher chance that something will happen to prevent you from taking care of your child. We need to be prepared for situations like that. Here's what you should include in your child's care plan:

- Their diagnosis and a brief description of what it is
- Their daily care needs (therapies or exercises, daily medications, skin-care, etc.)
- Things to watch for (warning signs for seizures, behaviors, possible infections, etc.)
- Accommodations (specific activities they should not participate in, different ways of doing things to accommodate their needs, etc.)
- An emergency action plan (what medicines to give, what hospital to go to, when to call an ambulance, etc.)
- A list of their doctors (include what their specialty is and the name of their nurse), therapists, etc. along with contact info for each one
- Any allergies your child may have to foods or medications

It may be helpful to keep one copy of your child's care plan with you, another at their school, another with relatives or friends who may end up caring for your child if you get sick suddenly, and another at home where it can be found easily. You can design the care plan yourself by just typing everything up on your computer or you can search for "special needs childcare plan" online and find templates that you can fill in with your child's information.

ADVOCATE FOR YOUR CHILD

I used to be really shy. I never spoke up, and I just took things as they came because I was too scared to say anything. That changed after Davy was born, and I had no choice but to speak up and fight for my baby. Thankfully, my sister-in-law, who is a doctor, helped fight for him at first because it took me a little while to get my feet under me, but now . . . don't mess with me when it comes to my kids' medical care.

Here's what you're going to need to know so you can be your child's best advocate . . .

If your child has any kind of special needs or illness, chronic or otherwise, they should probably have what's known as a 504 Plan or IEP at school. If you're not from the United States, they may be called something else and have slightly different functions and requirements so check with your school to find out what is available for your child.

A 504 is a health plan with accommodations and other information needed to provide your child with a proper learning environment. It's used when a child has a disability that interferes with their ability to learn in a general education classroom. In the United States, Section 504 of the Rehabilitation Act of 1973 is the law that allows for 504 plans.

An IEP is an Individualized Education Plan that is put in place when a child's disability requires the use of special education services. Unlike the generality of a 504, an IEP sets specific goals and how progress towards those goals will be tracked. It lists the services the child will receive and how often that will happen along with accommodations and modifications needed for the child's environment. The Individuals with Disabilities Education Act or IDEA is the law that applies to IEPs.

504s and IEPs and the services they provide are available to students who need them at no cost to the family. If you feel like your child is not receiving the services they need at school or are not being treated properly, you have the right to an advocate who can help mediate and resolve disputes.

Just like you may have to fight for your child at school, you may have to fight for them at the doctors' as well. I've run into my fair share of doctors who don't want to listen to me because I'm "just the mom." We actually left a world-renowned clinic that was supposed to have all the answers and be one of the best for care when they gave up on finding answers for Davy. Because they refused to acknowledge my concerns or run tests that I requested, things were missed that could have been very serious. During Davy's first appointment at the new health care system that we switched to, the doctor looked me in the eye and told me that I was the most important part of Davy's medical team because I knew him better than anyone else. When she said that, I knew we had found our new medical "home."

If a doctor isn't listening to your concerns or ignoring them, it may be time to get a second opinion or switch your child's care to someone else. A mom does more research than the FBI when it comes to their child's health, and doctors need to respect that, while they have many patients, we have just one (or more if several of your children have special needs), and we put our whole heart and soul into caring, researching, and fighting for that patient.

GIVE YOUR CHILD RESPONSIBILITY FOR THEIR CARE

One of the best ways you can help your child is by teaching them to take responsibility for their own care. Of course, the level to which they'll be able to do so depends on their age as well as their disability or special needs, but you know your child best and can determine how much responsibility they can handle.

For my kids, that means encouraging good habits with their medical care and giving them the tools to handle things themselves whenever possible. I've used sticker charts and rewards to help them remember to take their medications, and I hang up the exercises they need to do in the hallway near their chore clipboards so they can see them. I also put non-medication options for pain relief such as rice socks (for heating pads), and pain cream made with essential oils in a basket where they can reach them and encourage the kids to try those along with massage before asking me for an over-the-counter pain reliever. I talk to them about the appointments or procedures they have coming up and what will be happening during those. After appointments, we talk about what the doctor said and what, if anything, needs to be changed with their treatment plan. Whenever possible, I let them help make decisions about their care.

We also talk about what their conditions mean for them such as how it affects them each day, why they need to do things a little differently than other kids, and what it could mean for them if they don't take good care of themselves. I've found children's book about the things they live with such as Ehlers Danlos Syndrome, asthma, eczema, and amblyopia so they can understand them better and see that other kids have them, too. We've discussed ways for them to explain their EDS and other health issues to their peers and even adults. Basically, I try to give my kids ownership in their health which helps them feel more in control of it.

When you are talking to your child about their special needs or illness, make sure to pay attention to how they feel about it. Let them know that it's normal to be sad or angry about it and then give them the tools to deal with those feelings. I like to give my kids a Bible verse to write down and focus on and encourage them to pray about their feelings, just like I do when I'm angry or depressed about my chronic illness. My older kids also like to write in journals or write notes to me, but that doesn't work for all kids so figure out what your child responds to the best and work with that.

DON'T SHELTER YOUR KID

People with Ehlers Danlos Syndrome can easily injure themselves and dislocate joints, sometimes without even moving. (Yes, it's a unique talent, I know.) I'm painfully aware of the many ways my kids could get hurt because of their EDS. I would love to be able to wrap them in bubble wrap and keep them from playing outside or with other children who could injure them just by roughhousing a little, but that wouldn't do my kids any good. In fact, it would actually be bad for them, both physically and emotionally. Obviously, we take precautions and they know there are certain things they just aren't going to be able to do such as play football or play on the monkey bars. As much as I cringe inside, I encourage my kids to be as active as their bodies allow.

I also know that at some point, they're probably going to be picked on for being different or for having to wear braces on various joints. I can't protect them from that kind of pain either. The best I can do is give them the tools to handle situations like that.

MAKE SURE YOUR CHILD HAS A SUPPORT SYSTEM

When your child is younger, you're their main support system, but as they get older, they may need more than that. Finding a support group that they can attend is one way for them to get the support they need. Another would be to introduce them to another child around the same age who has the same condition as them. I've already made some connections in the EDS community so that if one of my children expresses a desire to get to know someone else with EDS, I have several moms I can talk to about setting something up.

Sometimes kids don't feel completely comfortable talking to us about their problems, and often, they don't want to burden us further. If you notice your child withdrawing or having a hard time handling the emotions that come with their condition, they may benefit from talking to a counselor or therapist.

DON'T FORGET THE SIBLINGS

When one child has medical problems of any kind, it's easy to get wrapped up in that child's care as a parent. However, we need to make sure that we're not leaving the healthy siblings out. Just as having a child with special needs is hard as a parent, it's also hard on the siblings. Often, they can feel forgotten or like they don't matter. Some may try to be as perfect as possible so as not to take any more of your time while others might lash out with negative behavior to get more attention. Every child is different and will respond in their own way to the stress of having a sibling with special needs.

Take the time to spend one-on-one time with them and sit down to talk about how their day was or their school project. Try not to talk about medical stuff and make sure they know that this time is for them, and they're important, too. Let them know that it's okay to want their own space sometimes away from their siblings and all of their needs, but also encourage them to spend time with their sibling so they can grow closer and get to know each other better. Let them ask questions about their sibling's needs and answer them honestly.

It's also important to make sure that your child has the support they need to cope with having a sibling with special needs. There are books, websites, support groups (both online and in-person), etc. that focus on the siblings.

Do you remember how having a parent with a chronic illness can teach a child things like empathy, compassion, responsibility, etc.? That also applies to having a sibling with special needs. There are positives and it can make for a stronger adult who can handle whatever life throws at them.

TAKE CARE OF YOURSELF

This is one of the most important parts of parenting a child with special needs. Have you ever heard the saying, "you can't pour from an empty cup?" That's completely true. If you haven't taken care of yourself, you can't take care of anyone else either. You have to make sure there's something in your cup to share with someone else. This is especially true when you also have health issues. If you don't take care of yourself, you literally cannot take care of your children.

Sometimes, I push myself too hard. I know I shouldn't, but I do and I'm willing to bet you do too sometimes. Oftentimes when I do that, I end up hitting a brick wall HARD and am unable to so much as lift my arm or stand up. At that point, I'm done. I can't cook a meal for my kids, I can't put them to bed, I can't even read them a story. More than once, I've called a friend or family member in desperation because my husband was at work and I was home alone with four young kids, unable to care for them. My cup is empty at that point because I didn't fill it up by taking a break earlier in the day when I should have or stopping to eat a decent meal instead of grabbing a can of soda, hoping it would give me just enough energy to survive until the kids were in bed. It is essential that I take care of myself and doing so means pacing myself and knowing when to ask for help.

TAKE CARE OF YOUR MARRIAGE

Did you know that the divorce rate for parents of kids with special needs is around eighty percent? Add a chronically ill mom to the mix, and I'm pretty sure that rate only goes up. We can get so caught up in taking care of medical needs for our child and ourselves that we forget that our marriage also needs care and time. Keep the lines of communication open and talk about what you're dealing with. If your spouse agrees to it, it would also be helpful to attend marriage counseling. People tend to think of marriage counseling as a last resort to try to save a marriage that's already falling apart, but let's compare it to owning a car. Cars require routine maintenance to run properly or you may find yourself stranded on the side of the road with smoke billowing out from under your hood. If you're driving and you start hearing a clunking sound coming from the left rear tire, you make sure you get it into a car repair shop right away or you may end up on the shoulder of the road with a car that won't go anywhere. Your marriage is the same way. It needs routine maintenance and immediate attention for even small issues or before you know it, it's in big trouble.

Even if your husband isn't interested in marriage counseling, that shouldn't stop you from going. I put off counseling for several years even though my doctor kept pushing me to try it. I figured that if my husband wasn't going to come too, there was no point. Finally, I hit a low point and decided to go for it anyways. I made sure my husband knew he was welcome to join me at any of my counseling sessions, but he never came. Despite that, going through counseling on my own was the best thing I've ever done for our marriage. I learned how to communicate better and how to work on myself instead of trying to "fix" him. Through the changes he saw in me and the improved conversations we were now having about our issues, my husband began to change, too.

The best thing you can do for your children is to love your spouse. Kids need to know that they have a stable home and are secure. If you let your marriage sit on the back burner so that you can focus on your kids, you're actually hurting them.

In my marriage, that means putting my husband before my kids. That can be hard to do as it's easy to get wrapped up in my kids' lives, especially when it seems like my full-time career is their medical care. The stress of caring for four kids with a genetic syndrome, plus my own health can be overwhelming at times, and I've had to learn how to lean on my husband for support during those times instead of lashing out at him. I've also had to learn to give him grace. He may not say much about it, but it's not easy having a wife who's sick all the time and four kids who have medical needs of their own. I need to remember that this affects him, too, and he's dealing with a lot of the same emotions as I am.

One of the ways that we keep our marriage strong is to have supper together every night. My husband works full-time plus he farms with his dad and brother, so he usually doesn't get home until 8:30 to 10:00 at night. By that time, I've fed the kids supper and they're in bed (hopefully sleeping) so we sit down to eat together. We don't get the chance to go out very much because of his crazy schedule so doing that is like having a mini date every night because it's just me and him with no interruptions. Yes, it stinks that he hardly gets to see the kids, but as they are getting older, he's able to take them to the farm with him more often so they can spend time together. One time, my kids asked me why I don't eat supper with them, and I explained that that's Mom and Dad's time and that's very special to us because we love each other. The kids all thought that was a neat idea and were happy with my answer.

One of the most important things I've ever heard about marriage is that it's not 50/50. It's 100/100. Both people giving their all to the other one sacrificially is what makes a beautiful, strong marriage.

CHAPTER TEN WRAP-UP

- Be a good example for your child on how to live with medical needs.
- Focus on the positives of what living with medical needs can teach your child.
- Remember that we're all different from the color of our skin to our unique talents. Your child's special needs are just one more part of who they are. We all have weaknesses and strengths and we all go through hard stuff in life.
- If your child inherited their medical condition from you, don't feel guilty. Life is still worth living even when it's hard.
- Watch for signs of depression in your child and get help immediately if you suspect they have it.
- Being organized is essential when you're dealing with your child's medical needs, your medical needs, and brain fog/low spoons. Put together a care plan for your child so others can care for them, too, if something happens to you.
- You are your child's best advocate. Advocate for them at school and at doctors' appointments. Remember, you know your child better than anyone else.
- Give your child responsibility for their own care and well-being.
- Don't forget about your child's siblings!
- Don't shelter your child. Let them live life the best that they can.
- Make sure your child has a support system in place, whether it be you, a support group, or professionals.
- Take care of yourself and your marriage. You can't pour from an empty cup!

CHAPTER ELEVEN
PREPPING FOR MEDICAL APPOINTMENTS

THANKS TO MY SEVERE ASTHMA, I've spent a lot of time in clinics and hospitals since I was a toddler. I've been to hundreds of doctors' appointments (please don't make me do the math for the exact number), and I've learned how to speak up and ask questions when I have them. However, it wasn't until after Davy was born that I truly learned how to prepare for a doctor's appointment.

When Davy was three weeks old, I brought him to the clinic because he was crying when I tried to feed him, and he was not eating as much as he should have by that age. His appointment was with the family practice doctor at our small-town clinic who I had seen since I was a kid. I had even gone to her for each of my four pregnancies until I was far enough along to be sent to the OB-GYN clinic thirty-five miles away. While we were there, she listened to his lungs and was alarmed to hear how junky he sounded so she sent us straight to urgent care. I scrambled to find a babysitter for my three older kids and neglected to grab any supplies such as snacks, my phone charger, etc. before driving the forty-five minutes to Urgent Care with Davy. We spent several hours there before the doctor decided that Davy should be admitted because of how young he was. I scrambled once again, while praying my phone wouldn't die, to find someone to watch the kids overnight so my husband could come be with us at the hospital. However, just before we were sent upstairs to a hospital room, the doctor noticed a heart murmur.

That changed our plans again as the hospital we were at did not have the equipment to check his heart and so we were sent across town to the bigger hospital. When we arrived, an ultrasound was done on Davy's heart, and they concluded that he had a Patent Foramen Ovale or PFO heart murmur which did not require treatment as they were sure it would eventually close up on its own (it did, by the way). He was monitored overnight and then released the next morning since he did not require any oxygen for his rattling breathing during the night. Several times, I mentioned that he had been having a hard time taking his bottles lately, but between the doctors' concern for his breathing and heart murmur, plus the fact that the little stinker drank his bottles with no problems while we were at the hospital, my concerns were dismissed as just being a worried mom.

When Davy was released from the hospital that first time, we were told to bring him back if his breathing worsened. It didn't, but it never got better either. It wasn't until he was around five months old that he was diagnosed with Tracheomalacia which is where the trachea is floppy and doesn't open all the way when you breathe, cutting off airflow. Severe cases need surgery to correct it, but thankfully, Davy outgrew his and hardly has any issues with it now at the age of four. When he was a baby though, it made his lungs sound very junky and rattling, he coughed all the time, and he would often turn blue, especially when he cried.

Over the next five weeks, I took Davy to our family doctor multiple times for weight checks and to try to figure out why he was having such a hard time eating. Thankfully, she knew me and my kids very well and knew that I wasn't just being a worrywart mom. However, even she didn't realize how bad it was because I didn't know how to prepare for the appointments other than to show up and tell her that he didn't seem to be eating enough. Finally, I decided to track how much he ate during a twenty-four-hour period. By this point, nearly all my time was spent with a screaming baby in one arm and a bottle in the other trying desperately to get him to eat. Most of the time, he would take a few swallows and then pull away and start screaming. So the next time I took him to the doctor, I handed her the paper where I had written down exactly when he ate and how much for twenty-four hours. It came to a total of between seven and eight ounces for the entire twenty-four-hour period. He should have been eating almost double that much. Instead of increasing how much he was eating, he was decreasing and was now losing weight. At two months old, he weighed less than nine pounds and was losing several ounces a week. Once the doctor saw that paper, she realized just how serious it was and before I knew it, he and I were headed back up to the hospital to be admitted. This time he was there for nine days. My husband's sister is a doctor, and when she heard that her nephew was in the hospital and no one knew what was wrong with him, she immediately took time off work and drove several hours to come be with us.

It was because of my sister-in-law that I learned what questions to ask and how to advocate for my baby. A few days into Davy's hospital stay, she advised me to purchase a notebook so that I could track his weight, write down questions for the doctors, note down what they were telling me, etc. That notebook became my weapon in my fight for Davy during his first year. I also had to learn to speak up and demand things for my baby. That particular skill was slow to develop, and we relied on my sister-in-law a lot during Davy's first year to help us fight for him when the doctors were refusing to listen or take us seriously. I learned never to go into an appointment unprepared, but to write down questions, research extensively, and make sure that they went over every question with me before leaving the room.

All that practice in preparing is what helped me when I realized that I needed to figure out what was wrong with me as well. After spending years asking doctors why I had so much pain and why weird things kept going wrong with my body with no answers, I had pretty much given up on ever knowing. However, I was rapidly getting worse, and I knew it was time to actively start looking for answers. Unlike the many times I'd been to the doctor before, this time I knew that I had to go in prepared. The weeks before my appointment were spent listing all my symptoms, researching possible diagnoses and tests, writing down questions, etc. When I walked into my appointment (with the same family doctor that Davy had seen in his early months and who had gone to bat for him with the doctors at the hospital many times), I was ready. I handed the doctor a paper with my symptoms written on it, front and back. Her eyes widened as she read through it, and it was obvious that she finally realized that something was going on with me. She referred me to a neurologist who ran a bunch of tests that all came back normal.

The neurologist then referred me to a rheumatologist who was booked out for almost a year. However, while I was waiting for that appointment, I spent my time continuing to research causes for my issues and Davy's. On September 1, 2015, I posted a picture on social media of Davy's foot bent up to his leg which he could do because of his hypermobility. Someone asked if he had Ehlers Danlos Syndrome and so I added that to the list of possibilities that I needed to research. About five minutes into reading about EDS, I knew we had found our answers. I also saw characteristics of EDS in my two oldest children and possibly my third as well. That March, Davy had an appointment with his geneticist, and I came with charts of EDS symptoms, diagnostic criteria, and how each of us fit those symptoms. When I presented the information, it was like a light went on in the room. We left that appointment with an unofficial diagnosis for both Davy and me along with more appointments to officially diagnose us and to test my three other children as well.

So, how can you be prepared for your medical appointments? Here's a list of tips and tricks.

FIND THE RIGHT DOCTOR

It's not always enough to just call the clinic and ask for an appointment with the first available doctor. Most clinics now have a list of their doctors and specialties on the clinic's website so you can find out who is available for each department. You can then look for reviews online for each doctor. I've also found it helpful to ask in local Facebook groups pertaining to my condition if anyone has seen the doctors I'm considering. Find out what their experience was like but remember that sometimes even doctors have bad days. However, if multiple people tell you that Dr. Smith was rude and brushed off their concerns, it's probably a good idea to cross his name off your list.

RESEARCH, RESEARCH, RESEARCH!

Even if you have a diagnosis and think you know everything about your condition, the medical field is constantly changing with new treatments, tests, and medications. You will need to stay on top of the information in order to be prepared. I've actually told doctors about new treatments available that they hadn't even heard of yet and as a result, was able to try them (usually with success). Your doctor is one person and can't possibly know everything about every disease and disorder out there which is why it's up to you as the patient to be in control of your care and to know everything you can about it.

It's not enough to just type your question into the search bar and go with the first website that pops up. You'll have to learn to check sources and make sure you're getting your information from reputable sites. The Mayo Clinic website is a basic one to start with. If you want to go more in-depth, the US National Library of Medicine (nlm.nih.gov) has tons of resources and information. You can also look to see if the condition you have, or suspect you have, has an official organization with a website as they will often have lots of resources available as well.

Many doctors will roll their eyes and disregard anything you say if you start with "I read about this on the internet . . . " Part of advocating for yourself is knowing how to present information to your doctor. The fact is that your doctor probably sees a lot of patients who "self-diagnose" after reading something on the internet and oftentimes, what those patients have read is flawed and not an appropriate source of information. Make sure you stand out from the crowd. Show your doctor respect but know that you can disagree with what they say and respectfully present new ideas for them to consider. If you have information from a reputable site on the internet to show your doctor, print it out, making sure that the URL is printed on the page so that your doctor can read it for him or herself instead of hearing it second hand. That shows that you are serious about your research and make him or her more likely to listen to you.

WRITE AN OVERVIEW OF YOUR MEDICAL HISTORY

This is especially important if you're seeing a new doctor that you haven't been to before. A brief overview of your history can be quite helpful. Include your current and past diagnoses, the medications you currently take and their dosages, your current symptoms, etc. Once you write it up, all you'll have to do is keep it up to date and bring it to new appointments instead of redoing it each time.

TRACK EVERYTHING

Tracking your symptoms, pain levels, energy levels, eating habits, etc. can really help a doctor get a clear picture of what's going on with you. I've found that it's very helpful to bring written documentation of my health. Doctors tend to take that more seriously than if you were to try to explain things to them, and it also helps you remember things better.

KEEP A RUNNING LIST OF QUESTIONS

I have a note saved in my phone called "Questions for doctors" with a section for each member of my family. That way I have it with me when I'm at the clinic and can pull it out and make sure to ask all the questions I have. My doctor has gotten to the point where she expects me to take out my phone and start going down the list of questions I have. If your doctor doesn't take the time to listen to your questions and answer them, it may be time to find a new doctor.

Be careful to not overwhelm the doctor with questions, though. I try to prioritize the questions I have and focus on the more important ones unless the doctor has plenty of time to answer them. Doctors are often busy so don't expect them to sit there for an hour answering your questions. We need to be realistic and respectful of the doctor's time.

Many health care systems have online portals available now so it may be appropriate to send a message to your doctor with a question now and then as well. I've found that doing so has kept us from having to make extra appointments which saves time for my family and the doctor.

USE A MEDICAL BINDER

By the time Davy was six months old, I had compiled a three-ring binder of everything I needed to be prepared for his appointments and care for him at home. His doctors and nurses thought it was the best idea ever and many of them said they wished more patients would do things like that. Several of them encouraged me to digitize my idea and sell it as a printable, so when Davy was a little bit older and I could actually put him down to play instead of holding him all the time, I did just that. It's available on my website, www.sunshineandspoons.com, and comes with over thirty printable pages so that you can print whatever and however many of the pages you need.

DOUBLE-CHECK INFORMATION BEFORE LEAVING

Before you leave the doctor's office, double-check any information your doctor gave you such as new directions for a medication, follow-up requests, etc. Many clinics print that information for you on an appointment summary when you check out of your appointment, and you can ask your doctor to make sure he or she writes everything pertinent down in their notes so that it will be printed on your summary. If your clinic doesn't have that available, write everything down as soon as you can or during the appointment. If you can find someone to go with you to your appointment (preferably a responsible adult versus one of your kids), that is also a good idea as they can help remind you of things, both while you're at the appointment and afterward.

If possible, schedule any follow-up appointments before you leave the clinic and make sure you write them down right away in your calendar, whether you use a paper planner or the calendar on your phone.

YOU ARE YOUR BEST ADVOCATE

Remember that you are your best advocate. You know what's going on with your health better than anyone else. Don't be afraid to speak up for yourself and get a second opinion if necessary. You can do this.

CHAPTER ELEVEN WRAP-UP

- Find the right doctor. Look up reviews on the potential doctors before scheduling an appointment.
- Do your research, but make sure it's from reputable sources.
- Write down an overview of your medical history to bring along to appointments. This is especially important if you're seeing a new doctor.
- Track everything! Keep a diary of your symptoms to show the doctor.
- Keep a running list of questions you have for your doctors, so you don't forget to ask them when you're at the clinic.
- Use a medical binder to organize your medical information and stay prepared for appointments.
- Double-check all instructions, follow-up appointments, etc before leaving the clinic. Bring someone along to your appointments if possible.
- Remember that you are your best advocate!

CHAPTER TWELVE
PARENTING FROM THE COUCH

I RELUCTANTLY PICKED UP THE phone and called my mom to ask her to come help me. I knew she was busy with her job as director of the local library along with the bluegrass band she played in with my dad and one of their friends. She was the last person I wanted to bother, but I knew I had to do it for my kids. I'd already called both of my sisters and neither one was able to drop their busy lives to come take care of their poor, sick sister. I even called a few friends, but they were busy, too. With each call that I made, I lost a little more of my energy and will to live. My mom was my final call and last hope that day.

I'd awakened feeling fine and ready to take on the world. I wrote up a lengthy to-do list for the day and optimistically began to tackle it while the kids ate their breakfast and spilled milk and cereal all over my previously clean vinyl tablecloth. That was fine. I could clean it up, no problem. But I missed the flashing red lights and sirens screaming in my head to "slow down!!" and before I knew it, I had slammed right into a brick wall, dropping me so hard that all I could do was lay on the couch and feebly lift my head. Even talking on the phone felt like too much work, but I had four young kids at home all day and no way to take care of them. My husband was at work for the next ten hours and was as inaccessible to me as if he were on the moon.

My last call paid off. My mom said that she could come over and help me out with lunchtime for the kids and then stay for at least a few hours. While I waited for her to arrive, I turned to Netflix to parent for me so I could lay on the couch uselessly, sipping Gatorade and mindlessly scrolling down my newsfeed on Facebook to see how awesome all my friends were at parenting and life in general. The kids were thrilled because they were getting to watch their favorite shows early in the morning, and Grandma was on her way. Despite their excitement and my mom's willingness to clear her schedule for a while so she could take care of us, I felt like a failure. This wasn't the first time this had happened, and it definitely wouldn't be the last either. What kind of mom couldn't even take care of her own kids?

As my (amazingly awesome) mom cleared the breakfast dishes and wiped the last of the milk off of the table so she could feed the kids their lunch, I tried as hard as I could to relax so I could gain back a few spoons to help me survive after she left for the day. I asked her to get the kids in their pajamas at 4:00 in the afternoon so I wouldn't have to do it later and to put together something easy for supper that I could throw in the microwave to heat up before serving it to the kids on our finest paper plates.

After my mom left that day to go back to her job, the kids decided that they were going to become professional lawyers and argue nonstop with each other. I dug deep in my foggy brain and came up with an idea. "Let's have a dance party until suppertime," I said with as much enthusiasm as I could muster.

I found a fun playlist on my phone and cranked it up while the kids burned energy jumping all over, and I cheered for them from the couch. When it was time to eat, I left the music going so the kids could keep dancing (and stay out from under my feet) until I finished heating up the food and dishing it out for them. Once the food was on the table, I switched my phone over to an episode of *Adventures in Odyssey* to keep them all quiet and still while they ate, thus cutting down on the amount of food spilled on my table and floor.

After supper, we still had an hour to kill before bedtime, so everyone grabbed their blankets and pillows and made themselves comfortable on the living room floor (except for me, I was comfy on the couch), and we had a reading party with cookies and books. The oldest two kids read to the younger two, and they all snuggled up beside me while I read a few out loud as well. When it was time for bed, I directed them to stack the books up and lug their bedding back to their rooms. Then I gave them each a task to complete their bedtime routine with instructions to report back to me when they were finished so I could give them their next assignment, being careful to rotate them so I didn't have three kids trying to go potty all at once. Once hugs and kisses had been distributed all around, teeth were all brushed, last gulps of water for my dry, thirsty children had been gulped, and everyone had been administered their nightly medication for asthma, eczema, allergies, etc., I tucked them all in, and returned to my throne on the couch—exhausted.

Do you see what I did there? To survive my "spoonless" day; I asked for help, came up with creative, non-messy ways to entertain the kidlets and keep them out of trouble, and somehow survived until bedtime. From my perspective, it seemed like a wasted day, but to my kids, I was the awesome mom who called Grandma, let them watch TV, eat off paper plates, and did some fun activities with them.

When you have a chronic illness, that means getting creative when it comes to parenting, especially during the times that you're stuck in bed or on the couch. You may be going along with a ton of good days in a row and then be viciously knocked over in a second. Or maybe you have more bad days than good days. No matter what, you're going to have to be prepared to effectively parent from the couch. This is particularly difficult when you have young children who need constant attention and care, but it does get easier, I promise!

As the expectations and needs change with the different ages and stages of kids, let's start with the first one and work our way up.

BABIES

Babies are fairly easy until they're mobile. That is unless they have colic or are high needs like my boys were. If that's the case, then my best advice is to do what you have to do to survive. Sorry. That's all I've got.

When my kids were infants, I had a "baby box" that I stocked with all the essentials for their care . . . bottles, bottled water, and formula for bottle feeding, disposable breast pads for nursing, diapers, wipes, diaper rash cream, burp rags, pacifiers, etc. That way I could easily carry it from room to room in the house and not have to run all over the house collecting what I needed for the baby right then. If I was having a low spoons day, I could just set the box next to me so I could take care of the baby from my bed. I recommend setting up your own baby box and keeping it fully stocked. In that same manner, always try to keep the diaper bag fully stocked as well. That makes getting out of the house *so* much easier when you're low on spoons.

You know those adorable little flannel receiving blankets that you probably got a ton of at your baby shower? Babies outgrow them almost right away, but they make awesome burp rags that can soak up a lot of baby spit-up. I found it helpful to keep some of these around, so I didn't have to constantly get up to find a new burp rag.

Make sure you're picking up and holding your baby properly to protect your joints and prevent pain and fatigue. If it's hard to lift the baby onto the changing table, change the baby on the floor. I hardly used our changing table and now it's a toy shelf because it was just easier to grab a wipe-clean changing mat and take care of it on the floor instead. Leaning over to lay a sleeping baby in the crib can be hard, too. Make sure your crib mattress is raised to a high level so you don't have to lean over as far, but then lower it as soon as the baby can sit up independently or stand. I'll be honest, there were times, I sat in the rocking chair through my baby's full nap because I knew I couldn't safely lay him or her in the crib while they were sleeping. Do what you've got to do to take care of both of you properly.

TODDLERS AND PRESCHOOLERS

If you have toddlers, this whole situation gets a little stickier (probably literally). Now you have to figure out how to preserve your spoons while keeping the toddler from flushing all of their toys down the toilet and smearing an entire jar of peanut butter on the living room carpet. It takes a toddler approximately 4.2 seconds to destroy a whole room and personally, I think this is the toughest stage, hands down.

One of the best things I found for dealing with toddlers and preschoolers was to limit the space they had access to. Close off rooms that they don't need to be in and use child proof doorknob covers. Use baby gates to block off rooms that don't have doors. I used to put the baby gate about six inches off the floor to make it higher so they couldn't climb over it while leaving just enough space beneath it that they couldn't crawl under it either.

Limit the number of toys that are out at any given time to cut down on messes. The less stuff kids have access to, the less of a mess they can make. You can do this by downsizing the amount of toys you have or by boxing them up to store in another room where the kids can't reach them. The benefit to doing that is that you can rotate the boxes and keep them occupied longer because toys they haven't played with in a while are basically new to them.

Instead of picking your toddler up when he or she wants to be held, sit down on the couch and have them crawl onto your lap. Teach them that Mommy can't always pick them up and that's okay because you can always sit together and cuddle.

Read your child books about having a mom who's sick. This can help them understand the situation better and learn to deal with it appropriately. Here are a few of our favorites:

- *Mommy Can't Dance* by Katie Carone
- *How Many Marbles Do YOU Have?: Helping Children Understand The limitations of Those With Chronic Fatigue Syndrome and Fibromyalgia* by Melinda Malott
- *Why Does Mommy Hurt?: Helping Children Cope with the Challenges of Having a Caregiver with Chronic Pain, Fibromyalgia, or Autoimmune Disease* by Elizabeth M. Christy

- *Mommy Has to Stay In Bed* by Annette Rivlin-Gutman
- *When Mommy Is Sick* by Ferne Sherkin-Langer
- *Ravyn's Doll* by Melissa Swanson

My kids don't nap anymore, but that doesn't change the fact that we still have rest time every day. Even though it's mostly so I can rest for a while, it also seems to benefit them as well and give them a reset for the rest of the day if they were a little grouchy or off somehow. When it's rest time, I set a timer for one hour. The kids are allowed to read or play quietly in their beds, but they have to be quiet and they have to stay in their beds. If they disobey either of those rules, I start the timer over again. After a few times of re-starting the timer, they learned that disobedience meant a longer rest time and now they follow the rules pretty well.

Believe it or not, there are lots of ways to play and interact with your kids when you're stuck in bed or on the couch.

- This one's kind of a no-brainer but read books together.
- Play "fetch" with your child. Seriously, toddlers love this, and it keeps them busy for quite a while.
- Play "doctor" with you as the patient (I know, right?) and your child as the doctor. All you have to do is lay there while they listen to your heart and pretend to give you shots.
- Keep a box of small toys near your bed and pull it out for a special treat to play with right next to you. You can even join in if you're up to it.
- Play peek-a-boo.
- Give them a bag of assorted pom-poms and ask them to hand you all of the big ones or all of the green ones.

For days when you don't have enough spoons to even do any of those things, or when you need to close your eyes for a few minutes (cautiously, of course since there are small children around), here are a few activities your child can do to keep busy and hopefully out of trouble!

Put together five or six themed busy boxes. For instance, you could create a music box with some fun shakers and other instruments that are made for toddlers or, you could put together a dinosaur-themed box with toy dinosaurs, playdough to make dino prints, and a dinosaur matching game. A nature box with rocks, sticks, and other things from outdoors would also be a big hit with kids. Just make sure they're past the stage where they put everything in their mouths. You could even put together boxes of random small toys and activities such as coloring books and crayons if you'd like. For more suggestions, type "busy boxes for kids" into your search engine and a whole list of blog posts and websites will pop up with ideas for you.

Hang a huge piece of paper up on the wall or tape it over the table and let the kids go to town on it with crayons or, if you're really daring, markers. Butcher paper works great for this. If your kids want to save their artwork, take pictures of it before tossing it while they're in bed asleep.

Give your child a page of stickers and tell them they can use the whole thing up, but they can put them only on themselves. You can get cheap stickers at a dollar store.

Cardboard boxes are one of my kids' favorite things to play with. They love making trains out of them, decorating them with crayons, turning them into forts, etc. We get a lot of our household supplies from Amazon Subscriptions, so we get big boxes at least once a month, and the kids are always really excited when they see the mailman carrying one up to the house.

Keep some special toys put up where the kids can't reach and save them for when you need a few minutes of peace and quiet. Make sure the kids know they are a special treat that they can only play with quietly when Mommy is resting.

Give the kids some big blankets and tell them they can build a fort. They can build one big one together or they could even each build their own and create a little "town" in which to play. Let them drape them over the table if they want and play underneath. Forts can keep kids contained in one area and occupied for a long time.

When I'm having a really rough day, I declare it a pajama day. We all stay in our pajamas, watch movies, and read books all day. On those days, we have "smorgasbord" for supper which is where I pull out different foods such as crackers, sandwich meat, raw veggies, fruit, pepperoni, dinner rolls, etc. and lay it all out on the counter along with paper plates. The only rule for smorgasbord is that each child must take at least three different foods. That way I don't have to cook, and the kids think it's a special treat.

ELEMENTARY SCHOOL-AGE

Elementary school-age kids are awesome. Right now, I've got three kids who are in this age bracket, and I'm loving it. They're old enough to have real conversations, develop a sense of humor that goes beyond just slapstick, and they're becoming more independent.

Many of the things from the previous section on toddlers and preschoolers can still be used with this age group. You don't really need to limit the space they have access to anymore, but keeping toys to a minimum is still a good idea. The books I listed earlier about having a mom who's sick can be good ones for kids this age to read with you as well as they're often dealing with new emotions and feelings. I still do rest time, but I will probably drop it entirely once all my kids are in this stage. Even my ten-year-old still loves busy boxes although I try to change out some of the items for ones that are more suitable for kids who aren't toddlers anymore.

Kids this age usually still love drawing and coloring so a large piece of paper they can decorate is a lot of fun. I love seeing how they get more detailed with their drawing and will even write notes on the paper as they get a little older. They especially love it when I leave a little note or drawing for them to find. Forts are always a blast, and as kids get older, they can make them more complicated than before. Of course, pajama days are a big hit with any age group.

One of the best things I taught my kids was how to make a sandwich around the age of five or six. When Davy was born, Katie was just six years old, and honestly, she was my saving grace at times because she loved making sandwiches for her and her siblings. They ate a *lot* of sandwiches during Davy's first year.

For those times when the kids need to burn some energy, but you don't have any at all, host a dance contest where you're the judge. You can even make numbers to hold up and awards to hand out to make it official.

Board games are fun and by the time kids are in elementary school, they can play quite a few. Using a tray to set them up on can allow you to play while you're resting in bed or on the couch. For even more fun, encourage your kids to design their own board game. They can either create a new game entirely or use an existing one as a template or idea.

Kids this age still like to be read to, but the fun part is that now you can move past picture books and onto books such as *The Chronicles of Narnia* or *Anne of Green Gables*. Once kids get a little older, they can take turns reading as well. If you're not up to reading out loud, audiobooks are fun to listen to together as well.

Scavenger hunts can be a fun activity to do with your kids, too. Give them ten clues, one at a time, for common household objects for them to find and bring back to you. Whoever finds everything first wins the scavenger hunt.

TWEENS AND TEENS

Tweens and teens are becoming more independent, and it can be harder to spend time with them. But there are still ways to spend quality time with them when you're stuck on the couch.

Meet them where they are. Play video games with them if that's what they're interested in or watch a movie that they like. Other ideas for activities you can do with your tween or teen include things such as board games, puzzles, listening to audiobooks, etc. If you don't have any shared interests, it may be time to try out something that they like as a way to bond with them. One of the best ways to bond with your teen is to just listen to them talk without any pressure.

AND FINALLY . . .

The most important advice for parenting through the rough days of a chronic illness is to ask for help. I know I've included this in just about every chapter of this book so far but learning how to ask for help can truly be your saving grace when you have a chronic illness. They say it takes a village to raise a child and they, whoever "they" actually are, could not be more right. We all must work together to help and support each other during parenthood.

Be specific when you ask for help. Do you need someone to pick up your child from ballet class? How about asking someone who's heading to the store if they can pick up a few things for you? Or what about watching your kids for an hour or two so you can rest. If someone stops by and asks if you need anything, ask them to vacuum the living room or just sit with you for a little while for moral support. Social media is a great place to ask for help without having to worry about being rejected since it can be put out as a general request and people can choose whether or not to respond.

CHAPTER TWELVE WRAP-UP

- There are activities you can still do with your child or children even when you're stuck in bed or on the couch. You may just have to get a little creative.
- It's okay to let kids veg out in front of the TV sometimes. Don't beat yourself up about it.
- Your kids don't have the same perspective of your parenting skills that you do. A wasted day for you where you don't accomplish anything except for survival could turn out to be one of their fondest memories.
- Don't be afraid to ASK FOR HELP!

CHAPTER THIRTEEN

HOUSEKEEPING HACKS

IT'S HARD TO STAY ON top of housework when you have kids. Add a chronic illness into the mix, and you have a recipe for disaster. Literally. My house often looks like a tornado went through it. Dirty dishes piled in the dishwasher and sink, a mountain range of laundry scattered around the living room that looks like it's waiting for a preschooler to scale it and plant a flag, two shelves' worth of children's books flung across the floor like some jumbo scale version of fifty-two-card pick up . . . you get the picture.

I'm not an expert and my house is never spotless, but I've picked up a few shortcuts and tricks to housekeeping when you have a chronic illness that I hope can help you, too.

Okay, so here's the best advice I have for you . . . hire a housekeeper! You're welcome. I know that was exactly what you were looking for in this chapter. A housekeeper or maid service is at the top of my wish list so if you're looking for something to get me for Christmas . . . but I digress. Since I know that hiring someone to help you around the house may not be a possibility financially, how about I share my other tips with you, too?

LOWER YOUR EXPECTATIONS

First of all, you're going to have to lower your expectations. That stinks, I know, but if you don't, you're setting yourself up for a lot of disappointment and anger. Lowering your expectations doesn't mean giving up and just being fine with a house so messy you could qualify to be on *Hoarders*. It means being realistic and giving yourself grace for the days (or weeks or months!) when you just can't keep up. Whenever you start a job around the house, remind yourself that it doesn't have to be perfect, it just has to be better. Also, don't worry about pleasing everyone else. I like to tell people that if they want to see me, they're welcome to drop in anytime! If they want to see my house, they're going to need to make an appointment. I'm doing the best I can with what I have and that's all that matters.

PACE YOURSELF

Let your body determine how much you're going to do at one time. If you push yourself too hard, you'll only pay for it later so break tasks up into little chunks and take frequent breaks. If you tend to ignore what your body is telling you until it's too late, set a timer for thirty minutes or fifteen minutes or even five minutes. Break it down into whatever you can handle at one time. Work on just one task for that amount of time and then set the timer again for a break. Repeat as much or as little as you can and give yourself a pat on the back for whatever you were able to do, whether it was just picking up the forty-seven dirty socks off the living room floor (why in the world do kids take their socks off all over the house?) or dusting and vacuuming the whole first floor.

SET UP A CLEANING ROUTINE

Having a routine can help keep you on track around the house. I've used quite a few different methods for my cleaning routine such as FlyLady, Motivated Moms, and a variety of smartphone apps. I now use my own combination of the things that work best for me from some of the routines I've tried. My routine consists of daily, weekly, and monthly tasks. For example, daily tasks include things such as emptying and loading the dishwasher and doing a quick pick-up of the living room. Weekly tasks include things such as mopping the bathroom and cleaning the microwave. Monthly tasks are things like washing down the outside of kitchen appliances and vacuuming under furniture. You can find a variety of basic cleaning routines on Pinterest.

If you run out of spoons and aren't able to cross anything off of your cleaning routine for that day, don't beat yourself up. Just pick up where you left off the next day or whenever you're able to jump back in.

Even if you're not able to keep up with a cleaning routine or just don't feel like it's for you, try to do a little bit around the house each day. Little things can make a difference, even if it doesn't seem like it at the time.

TOOLS FOR SPOON SAVING

There are a lot of tools that can make cleaning easier for you and save you a few spoons. I don't use all of the things on this list, but the ones I don't already own are on my wish list for sure. All of the tools I mention can be found on Amazon.

A reacher-grabber can keep you from having to bend over constantly to pick things up and help you grab things up high without risking a fall off a wobbly kitchen chair.

Dust masks are essential if you need to avoid breathing in dust and cleaning supplies while you work. My eight-year-old wears one when he cleans his room because of his dust allergies.

A cordless hand vacuum is easy to use for quick clean-ups. I can't always lug the big vacuum out, but I can grab my hand vac and take care of a mess on the carpet. My kids love using it, too, and actually argue over who gets to vacuum.

Even better than a cordless hand vacuum is a robotic vacuum cleaner that does the vacuuming automatically and on its own. Just set it and go. I don't have one yet, but it's at the *very* top of my wish list.

A long-handled dustpan to use when sweeping keeps you from having to bend over or kneel on the floor to sweep up your dust pile.

If scrubbing your floors with a regular mop isn't working for you, make your mop do the work instead. A steam mop cleans, sanitizes, and dries as you go, saving you elbow grease and a lot of pain and fatigue.

An extendable tub and tile scrubber can save your back and other joints and muscles (such as my elbow which I dislocated while cleaning a jacuzzi at the B&B where I used to work) from having to lean over a tub or reach high in a shower to scrub it.

Washing dishes or even loading them into the dishwasher is too much some days which is why I always keep disposable dishes and silverware in the cupboard. Aluminum pans are also helpful for when you just can't handle scraping and scrubbing the pan after a meal.

To help keep the shower clean, fill a scrubber dish wand with equal parts of dish soap and vinegar and keep it in the shower. Once or twice a week, use it to scrub down the shower before you get out (or ask your husband or even the kids to do it) and then rinse the shower down.

CLEANING SUPPLIES

Choosing the right cleaning supplies is important. Certain products do much of the work for you, cutting down on the amount of elbow grease you have to use. Many people with chronic illnesses also have chemical sensitivities so natural products are a must for them. I keep a bottle of all-purpose cleaner and other cleaning supplies in each area that they are needed so that I don't have to carry them from room to room or run across the house to get something. If something is really stubborn, I spray it down and let it sit for five to ten minutes and that's usually all it takes for it to wipe clean easily.

All-purpose cleaners are my favorite because they cut down on the number of spray bottles I need to lug around. The one I use the most is Thieves cleaner from Young Living. It's safe for the kids to use and can be used on anything, even mirrors. Plus, I love the way it smells.

Vinegar and baking soda are also must-haves in my cleaning supplies because they're so versatile, they cut down on the amount of scrubbing I have to do, and vinegar is a natural disinfectant. The two can be used together or separately to clean bathrooms, kitchens, carpets, etc.

A lot of people swear by Magic Erasers, and I love that they don't require a lot of elbow grease and don't have a chemical smell.

When I had my first baby back in 2008, I discovered baby wipes. I like to joke that if it can't be cleaned with a baby wipe, there's no hope for the mess. I use them for quick clean-ups around the house and car. It's easy to hand a wipe to one of the kids for them to go clean something up. My youngest is (finally!) potty trained at the age of four, but I do not plan to take baby wipes off my regular shopping list anytime soon. My only complaint is that if you leave them in the car during the winter, they freeze into one solid chunk, but I guess that's a perk of living in the Midwest.

DELEGATE

You don't have to do everything yourself! Don't be a martyr and use up all of your spoons for the month trying to clean the house by yourself. Expecting kids to help around the house teaches them responsibility and life skills, so giving your kids chores is a good parenting move. Remember, you're not just raising kids . . . you're raising future adults who will need to be able to take care of themselves and function outside of your home one day.

There isn't one sure-fire way to get your kids to help around the house. Some people swear by chore charts, others love sticker charts, and some fly by the seat of their pants. For my family, I've found that it works best to shake things up and change our methods every now and then. Right now, I'm using clipboards hung on a wall in my hallway along with some decorated wood blocks and other artwork (thank you, Hobby Lobby for your awesome sales!). It looks nice but is also functional. Each of my four kids has their own clipboard and the fifth one is mine. I write notes to the kids and Bible verses on each of their clipboards along with their chores for the day. They can check their clipboards by themselves and erase tasks as they complete them. Eight-year-old Nate likes to write his own chores by himself each night which I love because it shows responsibility. Sometimes, I steer him towards a specific task that needs to be done, but he's pretty good about picking chores by himself. Along with space for chores and notes, there is also a morning and bedtime checklist on each child's clipboard which has really helped streamline and smooth the morning rush and the transition to bedtime.

I've noticed that my definition of clean and my kids' definition are not the same thing. Like, at all. So I wrote a list of tasks that need to be done in each room for it to be clean, such as empty the dishwasher, wash off the counters, sweep the floor, etc. in the kitchen and fold throw blankets, pick up toys, etc. in the living room. I also included a second list of "extra" tasks that need to be done occasionally, but not every day such as vacuuming under the couch cushions, washing the trash can, etc. I laminated the lists and can easily hand one to a child along with a dry erase marker so they can mark off jobs as they accomplish them.

But what if your kids are too young to help around the house? Well, believe it or not, husbands can pitch in, too. Honestly, I can't say a lot on this subject because my husband essentially works two full-time jobs and gets home late most nights. He's pretty much only around to eat and sleep so he is not available to help out at home very often. He tries to do as much as he can, but for the most part, I'm on my own at home. However, I have no idea what your situation is with your marriage, so I encourage you to sit down with your husband to discuss the best way to handle chores in your household.

There are other ways to delegate besides turning your family into your servants. Just kidding. Don't actually do that. But seriously, other options include hiring someone to come in and do some deep cleaning once a month or maybe once a week. If you can't afford a housekeeping service, teenagers are often looking for ways to make an extra $20.

LAUNDRY HACKS

Laundry deserves its own section, for sure. It's the one thing I can never seem to get ahead of or catch up on for even one day. Once upon a time, I had a system and could stay on top of washing, folding, and putting it away. But then I had a few more kids—one of whom was medically complex—and my health started to decline, and before I knew it, we were buried under a mountain of laundry with no clean socks to wear. Over the last three or four years, I've learned to make small changes in how I tackle laundry.

Use a rolling laundry basket to move your laundry around. It's way easier than carrying heavy baskets.

Stop standing in front of the ironing board and ditch the iron. Dampen the clothes that are wrinkled and throw them in the dryer for ten minutes or throw a wet towel in with them to do the same thing. When you pull them out, they'll be fresh and wrinkle-free. Side-note . . . this does not work if you forget to take them back out for two days.

Some people swear by the one-load-a-day system of doing laundry, and others prefer to do it all on one day. I tend to skip back and forth between those two methods. My goal is to do a different type of laundry each day from start to finish. On Monday, it's all of the kids' clothes. Tuesday it's my clothes, Wednesday is all the towels, and Thursday is for Hubby's chore clothes. That system works pretty well for me *unless* we have a day full of doctor appointments (which happens at least once a week) or I have a day where I can barely get out of bed, let alone be productive. So, when that happens, I switch to the DO-IT-ALL method where I run the washer and dryer all day like a slave driver and just get it all done. Then, the next day (or month, whatever), the kids and I spend quality time together folding the laundry and putting it away. Figure out what works for your family and don't be afraid to switch it up.

Teach your kids how to fold laundry. They may not do a great job at first, but that's okay. They have to start somewhere. I sort the laundry into a pile for each child, give them each a basket and have them fold it. Four-year-old Davy still needs help, but he's learning and loves being like the big kids. Even though he can't figure out how to fold a shirt yet, he can fold washcloths and hand towels. When they have their laundry folded, they can push their basket into their room to put it away. It also helps to label their dresser drawers, so they know where to put their clothes. You can find special stickers on Amazon or just use masking tape to mark the drawers.

If you sort your laundry, you can get a laundry hamper with sections so that laundry can be presorted and save you time and energy when it's time to throw it in the washing machine. Or you can be like me and not sort it at all (sorry, Mom!).

You can cut down on laundry by downsizing to minimalist wardrobes for your whole family. Less clothes means less laundry. That means going through all your family's clothes to get rid of the extras and just keeping the basics and enough to get to the next laundry day. I know others who have had success with doing so, but personally, that means that we run out of clean clothes a lot since I can't guarantee that I'll be able to get laundry done by a certain day.

It never fails. Your kid forgets to tell you that their uniform is in the wash until ten minutes before they need it. This is where an "Emergency" laundry basket comes in handy. For uniforms and other pieces of clothing that will be needed again for a certain date, have everyone throw them in the emergency basket. Whenever you get the chance to do laundry, throw the emergency basket in first. Add other clothes to the washer if it's not a full load.

If laundry baskets are too hard to carry and a rolling basket is out of the question, thanks to stairs or some other obstacle, full-size reusable shopping bags work great for moving the laundry around. Just don't use them for groceries after that.

If it's hard for you to lift anything heavy, switch to laundry detergent pods. That way, you can just grab one out of the bag and throw it in the washer. Just make sure to keep them out of reach of the kids.

You can save spoons when folding laundry by not folding certain things such as underwear and pajamas. I grew up folding underwear and when I started having kids, I realized that I'm more concerned that everyone is wearing clean underwear than if it's wrinkled. So I stopped folding it and never looked back.

Folding laundry can be a boring job which is why I like to wait until the kids are in bed before turning on Netflix and sitting down in the middle of the living room floor to get it all folded. It goes a lot faster if I watch one of my favorite shows while I'm doing it!

I know this isn't possible for everyone, but if it is, consider installing a washer and dryer on the same floor as the bedrooms. For me, the hardest part of laundry is lugging it up and down the basement stairs. When my in-laws remodeled their upstairs bathroom, my mother-in-law insisted on putting a laundry area in there, too. She's a genius. I plan on moving our washer and dryer upstairs into one of the kids' rooms someday when we're empty nesters.

DECLUTTERING/ORGANIZING

Being organized is important for any mom, but when you're also dealing with a chronic illness, it's pretty much a necessity. Decluttering is a necessity, too, since belongings such as toys, books, clothes, magazines, random papers, etc. tend to multiply like rabbits and threaten to take over your house. Remember, the more stuff you own, the more stuff you have to take care of. Here are some of my favorite tips for staying organized.

Because I insist on feeding my children three to eleven times a day, they keep growing and so occasionally I notice that one of them is wearing a pair of pants that are beginning to resemble capris or their shirt has turned into a belly shirt. Usually, this is after they've worn said clothing for a long enough time (about four seconds by my estimation) to spill approximately eight different things on it so into the wash it goes. Unfortunately, by the time it comes back out, I've completely forgotten that it was too small so back into their dresser drawer it goes only to be noticed once again when it's in need of another wash. And the cycle continues. That is, unless I stick a safety pin in it somewhere where I'll notice it while folding. When I see a safety pin, I toss it in the inevitably growing pile of hand-me-downs and donations.

Every few years or so, I notice that my closet is getting a little too full. When that happens, I turn all my hangers so that they're facing the "wrong" direction. After about a month or two, anything that is still hanging the wrong way goes into the donation bag that lives in the corner of my room until it's full, at which point, it moves into the trunk of my minivan and lives there for another six months or so before I remember to drop it off at the thrift store.

I've found that it's best to declutter and organize as I go, but often that doesn't happen and the next thing I know, I can't get to my keyboard because of the piles of papers on my desk, the kids' toys are threatening a hostile takeover from the toy corner in the living room, and the pile of kids' clothes that needs to be sorted between hand-me-down, donate, or sell has grown to an astronomical size. So, every once in a while, I grab a trash bag and run around the house filling it up with things to donate. When I'm done, I don't look in the bag at all. I just tie it up and put it directly in my trunk with the other donations bags that are residing there. Alternately, you can also set a timer for five minutes and do the same type of thing to get some decluttering done quickly.

The one in, one out rule is a great way to keep things from building up. Even kids can understand the concept of receiving something new and sending something old on to someone else. Sometimes, my kids aren't sure they want to let something go, but after a talk about how we can share things with others and bless them with it, too, they're usually pretty game.

Some tools I like to use for organizing are Command hooks. I love that they also come in a Velcro version now. I also utilize a lot of baskets, both decorative and of the laundry variety, to hold things such as throw blankets in the living room, remote controls, and mail. Muffin tins are great for organizing paper clips, thumbtacks, etc.

You know all those papers that you can't throw out? Pictures that the kids drew, little notes, birthday cards, school papers, etc. . . . what do you do with them? When I was still in high school, I started collecting memories like those in a clear plastic storage tub with a lid that I decorated with bumper stickers. I still pop little mementos and other things in the bin and occasionally sit on the floor next to it and go through it, reliving fun times with friends and family. After my kids were born, I bought each of them a storage tub as well and wrote their names on each one so I could collect their memories for them to go through when they get older.

This is something I haven't done yet, but someone I know did it, and I thought it was such an awesome idea that I just have to include it here. If you screw wheels (easily found at any home improvement store) onto the bottom of an old dresser drawer, it makes a perfect under-the-bed storage option.

When it comes to getting rid of stuff, you have three options . . . sell it, donate it, or throw it away. If the item is broken, ripped, or in some other way useless, it needs to be thrown away. I tend to donate most things to local thrift stores, but there are some things I sell on Facebook Buy/Sell groups such as big lots of outgrown kids' clothes (example: $30 for a garbage bag full of size 3T girl's clothes). Selling them in lots saves me the spoons I would have to use to photograph each piece of clothing individually to sell. We don't have much for services around where I live because we're pretty much in the boonies (no take-out and hardly any restaurants. Ugh, first-world problems), but I've heard that some thrift store places will actually allow you to schedule a pick-up of your donations which is a huge help if you can't lug heavy bags and furniture around.

This section wouldn't be complete without addressing the organization of medical-related paraphernalia and information. In our family, four of us have asthma, allergies, and eczema and five of us are EDS zebras who use a lot of pain relief options, which means that our medicine cabinet is overflowing. In order to keep things straight, I separated the first-aid supplies into a basket on top of the fridge (where the kids can reach it with the aid of a kitchen stool) and then organized the prescription and over-the-counter medications along with the vitamins into the type of relief they offer. There's a bag for cold and flu meds, another for allergy medications, one more for pain relief, another for vitamins, and so on. Another box contains five Ziploc bags, one for each of us with our prescription medications ready to go. When I come home with our monthly pharmacy haul (seriously, the pharmacist always pulls out the big white bags when they see me coming), it's easy to pull the box out and drop the meds into the appropriate Ziploc bag.

I also use medical binders to organize our medical information. After Davy was born, I realized pretty quickly that having a medically complex child meant having to be extremely detailed with his doctors. I used a three-ring binder to organize his medical history with places to write questions for his doctors, reminders for appointments that needed to be scheduled, medications he was on, his daily symptoms, etc. I brought it to every one of his appointments, and his doctors and nurses loved it. Several of them suggested that I turn it into a printable and sell it online so others could use it, too. So, I redesigned it into pdfs and added a ton of pages for every need I could possibly think of. By the time I was done, I had over thirty pages. It's my top seller on my website, www.sunshineandspoons.com, and I've gotten tons of positive feedback on it. If you don't want to use a three-ring binder, there are apps out there that can also help you get organized and keep track of your medical information.

MAKE IT FUN

Cleaning doesn't have to be a drag. There are lots of ways to make it fun for you and your family. My kids like it when I set the timer so they can have a race to see who can get the most cleaned up before it goes off. This works great when they're cleaning their rooms. Sometimes I'll break them up into teams (which is why I am an advocate of having an even number of kids—haha) and have them work on different sections of the house. Every once in a while, when the laundry has gotten out of control, I let them watch a movie while we all fold together. However, that does involve a significant amount of reminding them to keep their hands moving instead of just sitting there holding an unfolded shirt for ten minutes while staring slack-jawed at the screen.

I've found that I don't mind cleaning as much if I listen to music, audiobooks, or sermons while I'm working. It takes my focus off the pain and fatigue so I can accomplish a little more than usual.

OTHER USEFUL TIPS

This chapter wouldn't be complete without some random tips that didn't quite fit into any other section.

While you're cleaning a specific room, throw things that belong in other rooms into boxes, laundry baskets, or bags to be moved when you're done. That way, you're not running back and forth, and you can just grab the box and easily bring it into the appropriate room. Don't forget to empty them and put things away, though, or you'll just end up with a bunch of random stuff in boxes and bags around the house. Not that I'm speaking from experience, of course . . .

Use kneeling pads (the kind that are made for gardening) for when you have to be on the floor working on something. I even use one when I give the kids baths since kneeling on the floor next to the tub hurts so much.

On the same note, sit whenever you can while you're cleaning. Sit on the floor to fold laundry, sit at your desk when you're cleaning it off, sit on a tall stool when you're washing dishes, etc. Doing so will save some of your spoons for later so you can keep going longer.

Every time you get up to go into another room, see if there's something you can take with you. Things like books that go in a kid's room, a towel that needs to go back in the bathroom, a glass that should be in the kitchen, etc.

CHAPTER THIRTEEN WRAP-UP

- Lower your expectations and don't worry about what others think.
- Take care to pace yourself so you don't run out of spoons.
- Figure out a cleaning routine that works for your family.
- Find cleaning tools and supplies that can help you save your energy for other things.
- Delegate, delegate, delegate!
- Laundry can be one of the biggest battles, but there are hacks that can make it easier to handle.
- Keeping things organized and decluttered can make your life a lot easier.
- Make it fun! Cleaning doesn't have to be boring.
- There are a lot of little hacks that can make cleaning a little easier.

CHAPTER FOURTEEN

LIFE HACKS

CLEANING YOUR HOUSE IS FAR from being the only struggle you have to deal with when you have a chronic illness. So, with that in mind, I compiled a list of life hacks that I hope will help you.

KITCHEN HACKS

My favorite way to cook is to dump stuff in a pan and throw it in the oven. My glass 9 x 13 baking dishes (I have four) get used *all* the time because it's the easiest way to make a meal for a family of six. The dishes that I do make on the stovetop are generally pretty easy and quick to throw together because I can't stand in front of the stove stirring a pan for thirty minutes. Also, anything I cook can usually be made in one pan to save on dishes. Just search for "one-pan meals" on Pinterest, and you'll get hundreds of options.

Did you know that you can easily doctor up a boxed meal such as Hamburger Helper or macaroni and cheese to make it seem more homemade? Just add a can of something such as diced tomatoes or corn or throw some cheese on top and bake it for a few minutes. I like to turn boxed macaroni and cheese into creamy mac n' cheese by stirring in a spoonful of sour cream and a handful of shredded cheddar cheese.

A slow cooker is also an essential appliance in my kitchen. The only problem I seem to have is forgetting (thanks, brain fog!) to turn it off in time so sometimes the food can be a little dark and crunchy on the outside. However, my husband recently got me a new one that I'm super psyched about because it has a timer on it. If scrubbing a slow cooker is difficult, you can get liners that make it super easy to clean. Just pull them out and throw them in the garbage.

Many times, when I cook, I double the amount of food and freeze half for another time. For instance, if I have to brown hamburger for a meal, I cook the whole package at once and divide up the extra into freezer bags for next time. If I'm chopping an onion, I do the same thing. A lot of meals freeze well, too, such as lasagna, shepherd's pie, meatloaf, etc. Aluminum pans work great for freezing an entire meal like that. When I need something to feed my hungry family but am completely out of spoons, I can pull a meal out of the freezer.

If it's difficult to stand in front of the stove or walk back and forth across the kitchen, a rolling office stool can help considerably. It gives you a place to sit and a way to get across the floor easily and quickly. I've used my rollator walker in the kitchen, but a stool would be a much better choice as it sits up higher and you don't have handles to contend with and, if you're like me, to catch on things and send them flying across the floor.

I struggled with my can opener for years, often having to ask for help to work the dumb thing because my hands did not agree with it. My sister eventually got sick of watching me fight with the can opener and the next thing I knew, an automatic, battery-operated can opener showed up in my kitchen. Seriously, I don't know how I didn't know that those things existed sooner, but it is now one of the most used tools in my kitchen. I highly recommend them for anyone who has a hard time opening tin cans.

Mixing and stirring things is difficult and painful for me most of the time and keeps me from doing much baking or cooking things that can't be combined with a few sweeps of a wooden spoon. Having a mixer makes such a difference and allows me to make a lot more food from scratch than I would without it. They're not just for baking. You can even use it to shred chicken.

Instead of cooking hamburger or chicken on the stovetop, throw it in the oven or slow cooker and then use a hand mixer or KitchenAid to shred or chop it up.

One of the best things I did in my kitchen was to rearrange it so that the things I use the most are easily accessible. I keep the kids' dishes (plastic plates and bowls) in a bottom drawer so they can get their own dishes and put them away by themselves when we're emptying the dishwasher. Kitchen appliances and dishes I don't use very often are put away in a high cupboard to make more room in the cupboards that are easy to access. You may have to rearrange several times before you find a system that works for you.

If washing and chopping fruits and veggies is tricky for you and there is a real possibility that you will end up with fewer fingers if you keep doing it, the extra cost for pre-cut food is worth it. Another option is using frozen fruits and vegetables which I actually prefer because the price is good, and they won't wilt and go bad in the freezer before we get a chance to use them up.

Cookie sheets or jelly roll pans can be hard to wash, but if you line them with aluminum foil or parchment paper, it saves a ton of time and energy on the clean-up.

Meal planning is a huge time saver and also means that unless we run out of something in the middle of the week (always milk and bread, am I right?), I can make just one trip to the store at the beginning of the week instead of going several times. I hit Pinterest up for meal inspiration and plan my weekly menu for the week on Sunday evening or Monday morning. It also helps when the brain fog is making me feel like I have cotton between my ears instead of a useful brain because I can just check my weekly menu instead of having to figure out what to cook with the eighteen random ingredients I have in my pantry.

SHOPPING

This is going to be a short section because there really are only two hacks you need for shopping.

First of all, order online! You can practically get anything online, and it allows you to shop around for the best price and use websites such as Ebates to get money back on the stuff you buy. Amazon Prime and I are best buddies. Walmart and Target are also at the top of my list with their free shipping (with a RedCard at Target and when you purchase a certain dollar amount at Walmart) and pick-up and delivery options. Even groceries can be ordered online now for pick-up or delivery.

Secondly, if you do have to go out to go shopping for some reason, don't be afraid to ask your doctor about a handicapped placard and then don't be afraid to use it if you need it.

HYGIENE

Hygiene can be a struggle when you have a chronic illness. Some days, a shower is out of the question or you're not able to brush your hair without pain in your shoulders and arms. These hacks can help you get through those days.

A shower stool can help you make it through a shower on days when you're not able to stand for very long. I recommend having one in your shower even if you don't plan on using it that day because slippery surfaces and poor balance/unstable joints/etc. do not make a good combination.

If you can't make it to the shower at all, dry shampoo and baby wipes are my go-to combo for a faux shower that I can handle while sitting down or lying in bed. There are no-rinse body wash and shampoo options available, too, if you want a deeper clean. If you need to wash your hair but are unable to stand in the shower, you can always do a quick wash in the sink.

If brushing your hair is too difficult to manage, consider getting a shorter haircut. I used to have waist-length hair but brushing it every day became an exhausting task, so I keep it about shoulder length now.

Mouthwash is an option if you're unable to brush your teeth for some reason. It's not as great as brushing, but it's better than nothing and it ensures that you won't knock your dear hubby over with your breath.

A wet/dry electric razor allows you to shave your legs while sitting on your bed instead of trying to balance like a dizzy flamingo in the shower.

Or you can use lotion and a regular razor to shave your legs. I started doing that about ten years ago and love that it moisturizes at the same time I'm shaving.

RANDOM HACKS

Use the alarm on your phone to remind yourself to take your medicine or head out for a doctor's appointment. My brain fog is so bad that I've used it for just about everything, including preschool pick-up, feeding times for Davy (he had a G-Tube and no hunger cues so we had to feed him on a strict schedule and yes, I would have forgotten to feed my baby without an alarm), and a reminder to start supper.

Keep a bag of emergency items in your car such as band-aids, pain relievers, braces, etc. I don't always have my walker with me in the trunk of my van since it takes up a considerable amount of space, but I keep a foldable cane in my emergency bag because it's better than nothing.

Use a pill organizer so you don't have to wonder if you took your meds that day. I like to use two, so I only have to fill them every other week. Pill organizers come in many sizes, shapes, and types. Some even allow you to pull out the section for that day so you can throw it in your bag if you're going to be leaving the house.

Sticky notes are my secret weapon. I write Bible verses on them and stick them on the mirror, use them to leave notes for the kids, and post reminders for myself. You don't have to limit yourself to the plain square ones that come in neon colors. There are a lot of super cute sticky notes available online.

By the time kids are about eight years old, they are able to take on more responsibility for themselves. One of the things I have my kids do by themselves is to pack their suitcases if we're going on a trip. I have a basic packing list saved on my computer that I can edit quickly to be tailored to the trip we're going on. I print it out, hand a copy to each of my kids along with a pen, and tell them to come find me when they're done. This saves me a ton of time and energy because packing for six people isn't for the faint of heart. I do recommend checking their suitcase though before you leave just to be sure they have the appropriate contents. The kids usually do a pretty good job, but every once in a while, you'll find a suitcase full of toys with maybe two shirts for a week away.

A lot of clinics have health portals online or through an app. I love being able to access notes from appointments, check for upcoming appointments, and send doctors a quick note if I have a question that doesn't require a full appointment.

A few years ago, on a Wednesday evening, Hubby was at work and the kids and I were at church. Towards the end of the prayer time, my throat started to tickle. Over the next few minutes, it got worse. Fast. I'd had that happen many times before, so I knew what was coming. My throat closes up with absolutely no trigger or warning. My dad called 911, my in-laws took my kids home, and I got wheeled out of church on a stretcher in front of everyone. It was *so* embarrassing. But even worse was when I was in the ambulance, and the EMTs had to ask me a ton of questions. My name, address, insurance info, current meds, etc. Ever try talking when your throat is closing up? Yeah, it's not easy. After that, I searched the app store on my phone and found a free app called Medical ID. I loaded all my pertinent medical information into the app and was happy to see that it could be accessed from my lock screen. That means that the next time that happens, I can just hand my phone to the medical personnel and be done. I showed the app to an EMT friend of mine, and she said *everyone* should have something like that on their phone in case of an accident.

And my last hack for living with a chronic illness . . . learn how to ask for and accept help. This one is tough but doing so can make the difference between falling apart and hanging in there. You can find a whole section on this subject in the first part of chapter two.

CHAPTER FOURTEEN WRAP-UP

- Hacks in the kitchen can make cooking a *lot* easier!
- Online shopping is the way to go.
- Hacks for hygiene can keep things, um . . . clean.
- There's a life hack for just about everything.

PART THREE

LOVING A SPOONIE

CHAPTER FIFTEEN
TO THE SPOUSE OF A SPOONIE

LIFE HAS A WAY OF throwing you some curveballs, doesn't it? You probably never anticipated that you would be married to someone with a chronic illness, yet here you are. I've written this chapter with the husband of a wife with a chronic illness in mind, but wives, if your husband is one who is chronically ill, this chapter is still very applicable to you.

Husbands, like you, your wife probably never anticipated that she would have a chronic illness. You'll both need time to adjust to your new reality and the best way to do that is to lean on each other and God for support.

Although I've always had health problems that restricted my daily life and activities, I didn't expect that my health would deteriorate to the point where I would be disabled by my thirties. My husband certainly didn't expect that either. It's hard on a marriage to have a chronic illness involved. It's that third wheel that just won't go away and can be very demanding.

When a chronic illness strikes, you have two choices in front of you. Will you pull away from God and your spouse and become bitter and angry or will you draw closer to both of them and move forward with your lives together? I pray that you would be able to choose the second option. If you have the right attitude, a chronic illness or other trials in life can make you and your marriage stronger. With that in mind, let's get down to the practical advice for navigating your life as the spouse of someone who is chronically ill.

READ THIS WHOLE BOOK

With the exception of a few chapters, this whole book *is* written for the wives. However, there's a lot of good information in it that can help husbands as you deal with having a chronically ill spouse and can help you better understand what she's going through. If you're busy or just not into reading like my husband is, I've included a summary at the end of each chapter so you can get a quick overview of the information in it.

THE FIVE STAGES OF GRIEF

The five stages of grief (denial, anger, bargaining, depression, and acceptance) were first used to describe what someone goes through after the death of a loved one, but they actually apply to anyone who's mourning a loss of some kind. When someone is diagnosed with a chronic illness, they must mourn the loss of the life they thought they would have, the loss of independence, and the loss of certain abilities. Your spouse may be the one with the chronic illness, but you're also mourning the loss of the life you thought you would have with them. You may find yourself going through the five stages of grief as well. However, grief is not a linear process and it's not the same for everyone. You and your spouse may be at different stages at different times. Maybe one of you will skip a stage completely or maybe you'll repeat a stage over again that you thought you'd already dealt with. Everyone is different in how they deal with grief and that's okay. Don't expect your spouse to handle it the same way you do. Just support her wherever she is.

You can learn more about the five stages of grief in chapter five.

IT'S NOT ALWAYS ABOUT SEX

God created men and women to be different and have different needs. This means that men need physical intimacy to feel loved and women need to feel loved to have physical intimacy. I've heard it explained that men and women can be compared to microwaves and slow cookers—men are ready to go at a moment's notice, and women need to warm up for a while first.

Sex is a very important part of any marriage and a way that God gave us to connect to each other on a deeper level, both physically and emotionally. Chronic illness can really throw a wrench into your sex life, though. Your wife may be in too much pain or have too much fatigue on a daily basis to even think about activities in the bedroom.

For me, I've found that it's not enough to assume that if it happens, it happens and if it doesn't, oh well. I have to make it a priority. Sometimes that means not folding the laundry after the kids go to bed. Sometimes, it means letting the kids watch TV first thing in the morning while we sleep in. My husband and I have to be purposeful about finding the time and making it happen. When physical intimacy is a priority in our marriage, we're both happier.

Be mindful of how your wife feels, though. Pressuring her to have sex when she's not feeling up to it can lead to her feeling like she's not good enough for you or feeling intensely guilty.

Sometimes, physical intimacy isn't possible at all thanks to your wife's chronic illness. You can use those times to build intimacy and closeness in other areas of your marriage. Recently, sex was not an option for quite a while thanks to my health. Yet I was able to be thankful for the experience as it brought my husband and me closer together in other ways. As a result, we had some good conversations instead about issues that we'd been having and ended up even stronger as a couple.

MAKE CONNECTIONS WITH OTHERS

You may benefit from connecting with others who are in a similar situation with their spouse. This could mean talking to your friend who also has a wife with a chronic illness, attending a caregivers/partner support group, or joining an online forum. Do whatever you feel most comfortable with and know that you're not alone in this.

CONNECT AS A COUPLE

Take time to connect as a couple without it being all about your wife's chronic illness or the kids. Find a babysitter and go on a date. Reminisce about when you first started dating or got married. Try to relax and just enjoy the time together as husband and wife.

DON'T FEEL THAT YOU HAVE TO FIX YOUR SPOUSE

Men often feel like it's their job to fix things. This is why it's so hard on them when they're faced with something that they *can't* fix.

Your wife's chronic illness is one of those things, and that's okay. As much as you want to take her pain away from her, you can't. Instead, focus on supporting her wherever she is and be her shoulder to cry on when she needs one. Sometimes, she's going to need to vent. Just listen to what she has to say, give her a (gentle!) hug if she needs one, and be there for her. That's the most important thing to her right now.

IT'S OKAY TO TAKE BREAKS

You're only human. You can't be "on" 24/7. That's exhausting and not sustainable long-term. If you're the caregiver for your wife, you're going to need breaks, and you're going to need to relax now and then. Even moms need breaks from their kids on a regular basis. Set reasonable limits and stick to them. Allow others to help with driving to appointments, picking up groceries, doing a little housework, etc. so that the burden doesn't fall completely on your shoulders.

AVOID CAREGIVER BURNOUT

Watch for signs of caregiver burnout. You may not even realize you're experiencing it until the pressure and stress has built up too much and you explode. The symptoms are actually pretty similar to the symptoms of depression. Irritability, loss of appetite, withdrawing from family and friends, feelings of hopelessness, etc. are all things to watch for. If you notice any of those signs in yourself or you feel like you're under a lot of pressure, talk to someone like a counselor or your pastor. Talk to your wife, too, and let her know what you're going through.

TAKE CARE OF YOURSELF

In order to be able to take care of your wife, you are going to need to take care of yourself. This means eating properly, exercising regularly, getting out of the house occasionally, taking your vitamins, etc. You know how the instructions on an airplane are to put the oxygen mask on yourself before helping anyone else put on theirs? That applies to the rest of life, too. It's not selfish to take care of yourself because if you don't, you will not be able to take care of someone else. Remember, no one can pour from an empty cup.

ASK YOUR SPOUSE WHAT SHE NEEDS AND BE SPECIFIC

It's not always enough to ask if someone needs anything. Sometimes, they're not even aware of what they need or can't narrow it down. Instead, notice the areas where your wife seems to be struggling and step in to lend a hand. Pay attention to when she's having a hard time emotionally and be ready to listen or give a hug. Ask her to give you some ways that you can help make her day easier and then follow through.

On the other hand, be specific with your needs when you're talking to your spouse as well. If you need her to show more physical affection, tell her, but do it kindly. Work together to make sure both of you are having your needs met.

BE YOUR SPOUSE'S BIGGEST SUPPORTER

Some disabilities are easily seen. Maybe it includes a facial deformity, a wheelchair, or leg braces. Other disabilities are what is known as an invisible illness. The person who has it may have their body that is literally falling apart on the inside or be in so much pain that they can barely move, but on the outside, they look healthy and normal. Your spouse may look fine, but they're really not. Invisible disabilities are tough to deal with because people who have them often face a lot of skepticism and criticism from their family, friends, and sometimes even doctors. No matter if your wife has a visible or invisible illness, be on her side. Stand up for her when others are questioning the validity of her diagnosis. Let her know that you're in her corner, and you're in this together. Your opinion matters more to her than anyone else's. If you believe in her, what others say won't hurt her as much. If you're having a hard time understanding her condition, go with her to one of her medical' appointments and ask the doctor to explain the ins and outs of your wife's chronic illness to you. Do your research and read up on it (but make sure your sources are reputable!). One of the best things anyone can say to me is "So, I've been reading up on your disorder, and I've learned a lot!" Be that person for your wife.

I know that between work and kids, it's not always possible, but when it is, try to go to your wife's medical appointments now and then with her. Doing that lets her know that you truly *are* in this together, plus it's not a bad idea to have someone sitting in on appointments with her to help her remember to ask any questions that she may have and keep track of what the doctor is saying. For appointments you aren't able to attend, ask how they went when you see her afterward. Sometimes, an appointment can be devastating, on a large or small scale, and she may need to cry or vent about it.

RESEARCH YOUR WIFE'S CONDITION

You can never fully understand what your wife is going through but learning about her chronic illness can help you better understand. As you research, be sure that you're getting your information from reliable, reputable sources. I have a friend who went online and researched Ehlers Danlos Syndrome after I was diagnosed with it, but he read only the first articles that popped up and then proudly told me that he had done his research and if I would only do this, that, and the other thing that I would be cured. In his eyes, I just wasn't trying hard enough to make myself better. That hurt. A lot. Don't be like him.

MARRIAGE COUNSELING

Statistics show that over seventy-five percent of marriages that involve a chronic illness end in divorce. In order to avoid ending up in that percentage, you'll have to fight for your marriage and find tools for combating the stress and strain that a chronic illness places on a couple. Counseling is not a dirty word, and it doesn't mean you're in the throes of divorce, desperate for that one last chance to save your marriage. It's a maintenance measure and a way to learn how to communicate effectively, which is one of the most important parts of marriage.

REALIZE THAT CHRONIC ILLNESS *WILL* CHANGE YOUR MARRIAGE

When I was diagnosed with Ehlers Danlos Syndrome, I didn't think it would change much about my marriage. But it did. It was a lot like adding another child to the family except it was much less rewarding and fun. We had to make some changes and adjustments to allow it room to exist because it wasn't going anywhere. For a while, it was the elephant in the room that needed to be addressed but wasn't as we kept living our lives pretending it didn't exist.

Change is inevitable no matter what and the sooner you accept that your marriage will be different with a chronic illness involved, the sooner you can both work on that adjustment stage. Your roles change and your responsibilities change. Maybe your wife has to cut down on her hours at work or is unable to work at all. There will probably be some trial and error before you figure things out and honestly, just as you do, you'll probably be thrown for a loop again. That's the way life is.

YOUR SPOUSE DOESN'T LIKE THIS ANY MORE THAN YOU DO

This really stinks for you. Your wife is not able to cook or clean anymore, she needs you to help with the kids all the time, she had to quit her job, etc. That puts a lot of extra strain on you. But as hard as this is for you, remember that she doesn't like this any more than you do. Probably even a little less. She's dealing with the guilt of not being able to care for her own family without help and maybe feeling like she's not a good wife or mother anymore. Plus, on top of the emotional strain, she is dealing with pain, fatigue, brain fog, etc.

This is not to say that either one of you has it harder than the other. A chronic illness doesn't just affect the person who has it and is hard on everyone in different ways. Be kind to each other and don't minimize what your wife is going through just because it's different than your experience. Talk with your wife about how her chronic illness makes you feel. Be honest and open. It may also be helpful to talk to someone besides your wife as well such as a supportive friend or your pastor.

REALIZE THAT YOUR SPOUSE CAN'T HELP IT

This is especially important if your wife has an invisible illness. She may look fine to you but believe me when I say she's not. She's struggling, and she's in pain. Give her grace and realize that she's not just doing this to get attention or to get out of doing work. She would gladly trade in her chronic illness for all the responsibilities she's had to give up because of it.

GIVE HER EXTRA GRACE ON HIGH PAIN DAYS

Just to warn you, your wife may be extra irritable and cranky on days when her pain is at high levels or when she's really not feeling well. However, I'm going to guess that you have already figured that one out on your own. While I'm not excusing her crankiness, I understand it. I get the same way, and I know it's not right and it's not fair to others when I act like that. Do you know what helps my mood the best, though? It's not the sudden relief of all my pain although that would work, too. It's a kind word from my husband despite me snapping at him for no reason. It shows me that he cares about my pain, and he cares about me even though I don't necessarily feel like I deserve it at the moment.

So, if your wife is extra grouchy, be kind to her. Chances are she'll be kind back or at least stop being as grumpy.

It also helps to know the triggers for her pain. A change in weather, cold weather or extra hot weather, stress, overdoing it, etc. can all increase pain levels. Be aware of those things and whatever unique triggers your wife may have as they can alert you to the days when she will be struggling more.

DIRECT YOUR ANGER AT THE SOURCE

At times, you're probably going to be angry and frustrated with your wife's chronic illness. That's normal. Just make sure you're directing your anger at the source and not at your wife. It's not her fault that she has a chronic illness, and she has to learn to deal with it just like you do. Measure your anger against the Bible to be sure that it's a righteous anger and not a sinful one. You can define that by determining what you're angry at. Are you angry at God for not healing your wife or angry at her for being sick? Those are both a sinful type of anger.

A righteous anger is one that is directed at sin and the twisting of God's Word. It's anger at the injustice of the world and how the innocent suffer because of the sin of others. The goal of righteous anger is a desire to change the situation and help others.

While you may be angry and frustrated sometimes, work on letting it go and moving on. If you let it eat you up inside, you're hurting yourself and your loved ones. Give it to God.

DON'T FEEL GUILTY

There may be times when you feel guilty that your wife has to suffer while you're as healthy as a horse. Don't. You can't change the situation and chances are she'd rather have it than have to watch you suffer. Just be there for her and let her know that you love her.

REMEMBER YOUR WEDDING VOWS

Even if your wife gives you a free pass out of your marriage, don't take it. She's probably struggling with feelings of guilt and worthlessness, but that doesn't mean she truly wants your marriage to end. When you got married, you made a promise to each other and to God that you were committed "'til death do us part." That is not something to be taken lightly. God isn't okay with us breaking that promise just because things get hard. Life *is* hard and the only way to get through it is to lean on Christ. Make God a prominent part of your marriage.

> And though a man might prevail against one who is alone, two will withstand him-a threefold cord is not quickly broken. Ecclesiastes 4:12

You and your wife are stronger together and even stronger yet if God is included in your marriage. When things get rough, that means it's time to draw even closer to God and each other instead of pulling away. Express your commitment to your marriage and to God. We can't choose our circumstances, but we can choose our reaction to them.

SHOW THE LOVE OF CHRIST

> Husbands, love your wives, as Christ loved the church and gave himself up for her. Ephesians 5:25

Do you see what that verse says about how you are commanded to love your wife? God says, *"as Christ loved the church."* Jesus **died** for us because He loves us so much. That kind of love is sacrificial and unconditional. It doesn't stop loving just because one person changes or because someone gets sick. It loves no matter what. If you're having a hard time with this, it may be time for some marriage counseling or maybe some extra time spent in prayer asking God to help you show sacrificial love to your wife.

CHAPTER FIFTEEN WRAP-UP

- Don't stop with this one chapter. Read the rest of this book so you can better understand what your wife is going through.
- Be prepared to go through the five stages of grief and remember that they are not linear, but often circular in nature. Also, everyone goes through them differently and that's okay.
- If sex is not possible, focus on building intimacy and closeness in other areas of your marriage. Be careful not to pressure your wife too much but let her know what your needs are.
- Connecting with others, either online or in-person, can help you feel less alone in your role as a husband of a chronically ill wife.
- Take time to connect as a couple.
- Don't feel as if you have to "fix" your wife. That's not your job and that's okay. Just be there for her.
- Make sure you get breaks from your responsibilities when you need them. It's okay to set limits.
- Watch for the signs of caregiver burnout and address them right away if you see them.
- Make sure you're taking care of yourself physically and mentally. No one can pour from an empty cup.
- Be specific when you ask your wife what she needs from you. Also, be specific when telling her what you need as well.
- Be your wife's biggest supporter. She may face a lot of skepticism about her diagnosis. Make sure you're in her corner.
- Research your wife's condition—make sure your sources are reputable.
- Utilize marriage counseling. It can be life-changing for your relationship.
- Realize that a chronic illness will change your marriage. Things won't be the same, no matter how hard you try to keep them that way. Accept that and move forward.

- Your wife doesn't like this any more than you do. Be kind to each other.
- Your wife can't help the way she feels. She may look fine, but she's struggling and in a lot of pain.
- Give your wife extra grace on high pain days. A little kindness can go a long way towards improving her mood.
- Direct your anger and frustration at the chronic illness, not at God or your wife.
- Don't feel guilty for being the healthy one in the relationship.
- Stay committed to each other. A chronic illness is not a reason to break your vows to each other and to God.
- Show your wife the same kind of sacrificial love that Christ shows the church.

CHAPTER SIXTEEN

WHAT NOT TO SAY TO A SPOONIE PARENT (AND WHAT TO SAY INSTEAD)

SOMETIMES PEOPLE MEAN WELL, BUT they say things that can be insensitive and cut you to the core. This is especially hard to handle when you've got chronic illness mom guilt on top of regular mom guilt.

I've had my fair share of comments that left me stunned and hurt despite the person meaning well (or not!). From the lab technician who asked why in the world I would ever have children knowing that I could pass Ehlers Danlos Syndrome on to them, to the "friend" who informed me that I caused my whole family to have EDS by vaccinating my children (um, that's not how a genetic disorder works . . .). People think they're helping, but sometimes all they're doing is hurting.

With that in mind, I put together a list of things never to say to a parent with a chronic illness. Some of them are a little tongue in cheek because I think we could all use a chuckle now and then. Also, every single thing on the list has either been said to me or another chronically ill mom I know. I wish I were kidding about that, but I'm not.

If you find yourself repeatedly struck by the urge to rip this whole chapter out to give to someone with certain parts highlighted and circled in permanent marker, don't worry. I've got you covered. You can find an abbreviated version of this chapter on my blog at www.sunshineandspoons.com/2019/12/

what-not-to-say-to-parent-with-chronic.html that you can share over and over again.

YOU DON'T LOOK SICK!

This is usually meant as a compliment, but it sure doesn't feel like it. Many of us have spent our whole lives trying to prove to our friends, families, and even doctors that we're not just faking this and that there truly is something wrong. Telling us that we don't look sick makes us feel like you think we're just faking the whole thing. And believe me, we wish we were.

Instead, try saying: You're looking good today, but how are you feeling?

I KNOW HOW YOU FEEL.

Um, no. Unless you also have a debilitating chronic illness, you really don't.

Instead, try saying: I don't know how you feel, and I'd like to understand better.

WELL, I'M TIRED, TOO.

Yeah, I thought I knew what tired felt like too before my chronic fatigue increased in intensity. Believe me, nothing can compare to this level of "tired." It's so intense that at times, I can't even lift my fingers to type on my computer.

Instead, try saying: I can't imagine how you feel. Help me try to understand.

HAVE YOU TRIED GOING GLUTEN-FREE? VITAMINS? ESSENTIAL OILS?

I've found the people who ask these kinds of questions are often trying to get me to buy a product that they sell. Sometimes, they're genuinely trying to help, though, and while I appreciate the thought, it's not helpful. I spend a lot of my time researching new treatments and possibilities as well as discussing things with my doctors. If there's something out there that I *haven't* tried, it's for a reason.

Instead, try saying: I can tell that you're working hard to research the best options for your illness.

YOU NEED TO GET OUT AND DO MORE ACTIVITIES WITH YOUR KIDS.

Two words... mom guilt. Mom guilt on its own is bad enough (am I doing too little for my kids? Am I a good enough mom?), but when you throw in a chronic illness, it intensifies significantly. Why would you want to add to that? Do you really think that I wouldn't **love** to be able to do more with my kids? Having to tell my kids no because of my chronic illness absolutely tears me up inside.

Instead, try saying: You're doing a good job as a mom. Can I take the kids with me on our next trip to the park?

YOU'RE TOO YOUNG TO BE SICK!

If only! Did you know that humans as young as infancy can have chronic illnesses or other diseases? There's no such thing as "too young to be sick."

Instead, try saying: That must be hard.

YOU SHOULD PLAY WITH YOUR KIDS MORE. IT'S GOOD FOR THEIR DEVELOPMENT.

Thank you for your wonderful advice. It never occurred to me to spend more time playing with my children. I would much rather lay on the couch and ignore them while I take a nap. Their development obviously means nothing to me. *Eyeroll.*

Instead, try saying: Your kids are blessed to have you as their mom.

YOU DID IT LAST WEEK, WHY CAN'T YOU DO IT TODAY?

Honey, I did something *an hour ago* that I can't do right now. Every day with a chronic illness is different, and sometimes, it narrows down to being different every hour. My body is very unpredictable, and I hate that more than anyone else.

Instead, try saying: Are you up to getting coffee with me today? If not, I understand, and, in that case, can I bring you a coffee?

AT LEAST IT'S NOT CANCER!

Oh. My. Word. Comparing illnesses doesn't help anyone. Ever. We all have trials to work through and each one is huge to the person dealing with it. For example, when I was still relatively healthy and had one relatively healthy baby, I thought that was incredibly hard (Example: my baby has an ear infection . . . this is the worst thing ever!). Now I'm basically disabled and have four kids with varying special needs. **This is hard.** But that doesn't negate how hard it was with just one child. Your perspective changes as your situation does.

Instead, try saying: I know it is hard right now, and I am here for you.

GET WELL SOON!

Here's the definition of "chronic" from the *Merriam-Webster* dictionary: *"continuing or occurring again and again for a long time."*

Do you understand what that means? I will not be getting better anytime soon. Telling me this makes me feel as though you really don't get what I'm going through, and that you don't really care to understand.

Instead, try saying: What can I do today to help you?

YOU LOOK AND SOUND HAPPY ON SOCIAL MEDIA, SO HOW BAD CAN IT REALLY BE?

Just because I am in almost-constant pain does not mean that I am never happy. If I waited until I felt good before I was happy, I would be miserable all the time, and that's not a good way to deal with this. Also, I only share things that I want to share on social media which means that you're probably just seeing my best moments. Would you really want to be friends with me if I did nothing but complain and exude negativity?

Instead, try saying: I am so glad to see that you were able to enjoy your day yesterday!

WHAT NOT TO SAY TO A PARENT WITH A CHRONIC ILLNESS (AND WHAT TO SAY INSTEAD)

I SPRAINED MY ANKLE ONCE, SO I KNOW WHAT IT'S LIKE.

Not the same thing. At all. I dislocate several joints just about every day and *pop them back in myself.* Also, sprained ankles heal. A chronic illness doesn't. No comparison.

Instead, try saying: I can't imagine how you feel, but help me try to understand.

YOU ONLY HAVE YOUR ILLNESS BECAUSE YOU THINK YOU DO.

Are you insinuating that I'm faking it and it's all in my head or are you telling me to be more positive so my chronic illness will just go away? Either way, **don't say this**. Seriously.

I know people think I'm faking it. I'm going to let you in on a little secret. I **am** faking it. However, I'm not doing it in the way you think I am. I'm actually faking being as well as I am. I work hard and push through a lot of pain so I can lead as normal a life as possible. I've had so many people tell me that I'm faking it that I even doubt myself sometimes. Do you have any idea how crushing that is?

Thinking positively can definitely have a good effect on mental and physical well-being, but no matter how positively I think, it won't heal my Ehlers Danlos Syndrome. I will still have pain, and I will still have defective genes.

Instead, try saying: I believe you. Tell me more about your chronic illness.

I COULD NEVER DO WHAT YOU DO.

I didn't think I could ever do this either. I used to read stories about people in situations similar to my current one and thank God that I didn't have to deal with that because I *knew* I didn't have it in me. However, that shows a lack of faith in God, and it turns out that you do what you have to do to survive when you literally don't have any other choice, and you do it with God's help.

Also, please stop painting me to be this amazing brave person who can power through something that most people couldn't. Sometimes, I'm barely hanging on and hearing something like this can make me feel like even more of a failure. If you only knew what goes on inside my head and behind the scenes, you would know that I struggle just like everyone else.

Instead, try saying: How can I pray for you today?

IF YOU PRAY AND BELIEVE, GOD WILL HEAL YOU.

Please don't turn God into a vending machine. That's not how He works. I can pray and believe all I want, but if God says no or wait, I am not going to be able to change His answer. Instead, I need to focus on what He is trying to teach me through my chronic illness. Do you remember Paul in the Bible? Remember how he had a "thorn in the flesh" (2 Corinthians 12:7) and prayed for God to remove it from him? God didn't. Instead, He allowed Paul to continue to go through his trial, knowing that it would strengthen his relationship with Christ.

Instead, try saying: How can I pray for you today?

YOU NEED TO EXERCISE MORE OR EAT BETTER.

So what you're telling me is that eating chocolate and sitting on the couch all day watching TV isn't the best way to treat my chronic illness? Huh. I had not thought of that. *Eyeroll.*

Instead, try saying: Will you tell me about some of the things you have tried with your chronic illness?

STOP BEING SO LAZY.

If only it were that easy. I watch other people my age and older keep up with their social calendar, work, go for walks in the evenings, and go camping with their kids. I would give just about anything to be able to be that active, but my body won't let me.

Instead, try saying: If you're up to it, would you like to go for a short walk with me? If not, I understand!

WHAT NOT TO SAY TO A PARENT WITH A CHRONIC ILLNESS (AND WHAT TO SAY INSTEAD)

I WISH I COULD STAY HOME AND NOT HAVE TO WORK.

When I was seventeen, I had to quit my first job thanks to my health. I cried for days because I was so crushed that I had to give up a job I loved and because quitting made the reality of my health hit me like a load of bricks. Right now, I'm a substitute at the local library and have to turn down a lot of hours because, after about an hour or two on a job that isn't even that physically taxing, I'm stumbling around like I'm drunk because my legs aren't working right anymore and practically gasping in pain. I love, love, love working at the library and had originally hoped to be able to go up to full-time when my kids get older, but now, I'm facing the realization that I will not be able to do that. Not being able to work makes me feel worthless at times.

Instead, try saying: Tell me about your hobbies.

IT MUST BE NICE TO BE ABLE TO PARK IN THE HANDICAPPED SPOTS.

You can have my handicapped placard if you take my disability to go along with it. I'm actually too scared most of the time to use my placard when I need it because people can be mean, judgmental, and forget that not all disabilities are visible.

Instead, try saying: Can I help you carry your bag(s) to your car?

I READ AN ARTICLE ONLINE THAT SAID YOU COULD BE CURED IF YOU WOULD JUST (INSERT RANDOM ACTIVITY OR WEIRD DIET HERE).

Neat! I didn't even realize that you were a doctor! Oh, wait . . .

My doctors and I have worked very hard to come up with the best treatment plan for me. Some random article you read on the internet that has absolutely no science to back it up isn't very important to me.

Instead, try saying: I read about your condition on (insert reputable source here) and learned a lot about what you're going through.

YOU'RE CANCELING AGAIN?

I hate having to cancel plans because of my health. Believe me, I would much rather go do something with you than lay in bed in pain all day. Please know that it doesn't mean that I don't want to spend time with you.

Instead, try saying: Can I bring a movie over for us to watch?

YOU GO TO THE DOCTOR TOO MUCH.

Yeah, I agree. I actually hate going to the doctor, but unfortunately, it's necessary for my health. If I stop going, bad things will happen.

Instead, try saying: Would you like me to come along with you to the doctor sometime so we can have coffee afterward?

GOD WILL NEVER GIVE YOU MORE THAN YOU CAN HANDLE.

Chapter Three in this book addresses this philosophy. I'd encourage you to go back and read it, but for now, here's a super quick summary . . .

You *will* go through more than you can handle, but God can handle it if you let Him. I *can't* handle this, and you saying something like that to me makes me feel like I must be a terrible Christian.

Instead, try saying: How can I pray for you?

To sum up this whole chapter so far, the absolute best thing you can say to someone with a chronic illness is "I believe you." Seriously.

Moving on from what others should or shouldn't say . . . what do *you* do when someone just isn't getting the hint about their insensitive words? Well, you actually have several options to choose from and you can use one or all of them, sometimes on the same person. Oftentimes, I go with a combination of the following.

LOOK FOR THE INTENTION BEHIND THE WORDS.

This one is hard, but sometimes it's the best way to avoid hard feelings on either side. Maybe your friend makes insensitive comments about your chronic illness but does it with good intentions. Maybe they truly care and want to help. If that's the case, gently explain to them that while you appreciate the sentiment, saying and asking things like that is actually hurtful and doesn't help. Be open and honest with them about ways that they can help encourage you.

IGNORE THEM.

When someone says something hurtful to me about my chronic illness, sometimes, I will just smile and then change the subject. Unfortunately, some people just don't get the hint, so you may have to move on to another strategy if this one doesn't work.

REALIZE WHEN IT'S NOT WORTH YOUR ENERGY TO ARGUE.

We all know a few people like this. They just won't let it go and there's pretty much no chance of them ever changing their mind on anything. When you run across someone like that, acknowledge to yourself that arguing with them is not going to help and it will more than likely end up using some of your precious energy. Answer their comment or question with something along the lines of, "I know that we don't agree on this, so I think it would be best if we talked about something else." Then change the subject, and if they bring it up again, use one of the other strategies to deal with them.

SET CLEAR BOUNDARIES.

It's okay to tell someone that you do not want to talk about your chronic illness with them and that it's off-limits. Once you've let them know that, stick to it because just like a toddler, if you give in once, they'll think it's okay to do it forever. Alternatively, you could also send them a link to a website that you know had reputable information about your specific chronic illness and tell them that you would love to discuss their suggestions and thoughts about your condition *after* they've read about it.

KNOW WHEN IT'S TIME TO CUT TIES.

If someone is intentionally hurtful or just won't let up with the insensitive comments and questions, it may be time to cut ties or at least limit interactions. You can unfollow them on social media (sometimes you can do this without deleting them from your friends list/followers so they won't even know), cut down on social interactions, "miss" their phone calls (caller ID really does come in handy sometimes!), etc.

CHAPTER SIXTEEN WRAP-UP

Things not to say to a spoonie, parent or non-parent:
- You don't look sick!
- I know how you feel.
- Well, I'm tired, too.
- Have you tried going gluten-free? Vitamins? Essential oils?
- You need to get out and do more activities with your kids.
- You're too young to be sick!
- You should play with your kids more. It's good for their development.
- You did it last week, why can't you do it today?
- At least it's not cancer!
- Get well soon!
- You look and sound happy on social media so how bad can it be?
- I sprained my ankle once, so I know what it's like.
- You only have your illness because you think you do.
- I could never do what you do.
- If you pray and believe, God will heal you.
- You need to exercise more or eat better.
- Stop being so lazy.
- I wish I could stay home and not have to work.
- It must be nice to be able to park in the handicapped spots.

- I read an article online that said you could be cured if you would just (insert random activity or weird diet here).
- You're canceling again?!
- You go to the doctor too much.
- God will never give you more than you can handle.

Things *to* say to a spoonie, parent or non-parent:
- You're looking good today, but how are you feeling?
- I don't know how you feel, and I'd like to understand better.
- I can tell that you're working hard to research the best options for your illness.
- You're doing a good job as a mom. Can I take the kids with me on our next trip to the park?
- That must be hard to deal with.
- Your kids are blessed to have you as their mom.
- Are you up to getting coffee with me today? If not, I understand, and, in that case, can I bring you a coffee?
- I know it's hard right now, and I'm here for you.
- What can I do today to help you?
- I'm glad to see that you were able to enjoy your day yesterday!
- I believe you. Tell me more about your chronic illness.
- How can I pray for you today?
- Tell me about some of the things you have tried with your chronic illness?
- If you're up to it, would you like to go for a short walk with me? If not, I understand!
- Tell me about your hobbies.
- Can I help you carry your bag(s) to your car?
- I read about your condition on (insert reputable source here) and learned a lot about what you're going through.

- Can I bring a movie over for us to watch?
- Would you like me to come along with you to the doctor sometime so we can have coffee afterward?

How to handle insensitive comments and questions:
- Look for the intention behind the words.
- Ignore them.
- Realize when it's not worth your energy to argue.
- Set clear boundaries.
- Know when it's time to cut ties.

CONCLUSION

EVERYTHING IN THIS BOOK IS what I wish someone had told me back when I was first diagnosed with EDS. Actually, I wish someone had told me all of this before I even had my first child, not that I would have necessarily listened to all of it at the time. That's why I wrote this book . . . to share with others what I wish I'd known from the beginning.

In case you were wondering, I don't always follow my own advice. I push myself too hard sometimes, refuse to ask for help even when I know I'm going to pay for it dearly, and I don't always remember to read my Bible every day. I don't expect you to follow this book to the letter either, but I hope you were able to find some nuggets of truth that will help you navigate your life as a spoonie. God bless you.

RESOURCES

Rest Ministries

    www.restministries.com

The Ehlers Danlos Society

    www.ehlers-danlos.com

Invisible Disabilities Association

    www.invisibledisabilities.org

Jolene Engle

    www.joleneengle.com

Hannah Wingert

    www.sunshineandspoons.com

ABOUT THE AUTHOR

Hannah is a wife of one, mom of four, and owner of Sunshine and Spoons. She has Hypermobile Ehlers Danlos Syndrome, asthma, Postural Orthostatic Tachycardia Syndrome, Mast Cell Activation Disorder, and an assortment of other conditions that make life interesting. She loves reading nonfiction books, writing, and chai lattes. Hannah lives in Minnesota with her kids, husband, and collection of braces and other medical devices.

For more information about

Hannah Wingert
and
Yet Will I Praise Him
please visit:

www.sunshineandspoons.com
www.facebook.com/sunshineandspoons
@sunshineNspoons
www.instagram.com/sunshineandspoonsblog

For more information about
AMBASSADOR INTERNATIONAL
please visit:

www.ambassador-international.com
@AmbassadorIntl
www.facebook.com/AmbassadorIntl

If you enjoyed this book, please consider leaving us a review on Amazon, Goodreads, or our website.

www.ingramcontent.com/pod-product-compliance
Lightning Source LLC
Chambersburg PA
CBHW070147100426
42743CB00013B/2836